HOSPICE,
A·LABOR
OF·LOVE

HOSPICE, A·LABOR OF·LOVE

Glavan • Longanacre • Spivey

CHALICE
PRESS
ST. LOUIS, MISSOURI

Cover: Scott Tjaden
Interior design: Wynn Younker
Art direction: Elizabeth Wright

Visit Chalice Press on the World Wide Web at
www.chalicepress.com

10   9   8   7   6   5   4   08   09   10   11   12   13

Library of Congress Cataloging–in–Publication Data

Glavan, Denise.
    Hospice : a labor of love / by Denise Glavan, Cindy Longanacre, and John Spivey.
        p.   cm.
    ISBN 978-0-827214-38-5
    1. Hospice care–Philosophy.   2. Hospice care–Moral and ethical aspects.   3. Terminal care–Moral and ethical aspects. I. Longanacre, Cindy. II. Spivey, John. III. Title.
R726.8.G56 1999
362.1'756 – dc21   99-30807
                                                              CIP

Printed in the United States of America

*To those whose stories we've shared
with you
and to those whose stories have yet to
be told,
we dedicate this book.*

Contents

Foreword

Death is an event that will touch every human being in this world. Many books have been written on the subject. Some are highly sophisticated volumes, while others are simple manuscripts. But all are intended to help us understand what death is about and how we can best deal with it when the time comes.

This book was written out of the heartfelt experiences of professional hospice caregivers from various disciplines. They have watched family members and patients grapple with the anguish and helplessness that the death and dying event brings with it.

This book is simply written, but every page offers words of wisdom that are profound and yet easily understood. There are explanations for the various changes that occur with terminal illness, and suggestions for practical ways to handle them. It includes a chapter on grief and bereavement so those family members can be assisted to go on with their lives after a loved one has died.

I found this book very useful, and it should be helpful for both professional and lay caregivers, as well as family members and all those who are facing either their own death or the death of someone they love.

Josefina B. Magno, M.D.
President, International Hospice Institute & College

Introduction

John Spivey

If you would indeed behold the spirit of death,
Open your heart wide unto the body of life.
For life and death are one,
Even as the river and the sea are one.

Kahlil Gibran[1]

It is one thing for philosophers to speak loftily, if not beautifully, about life and death being one. But for many of us, it is just so many words...until we are actually faced with death. And when we are, we find ourselves confronted with emotions we have kept safely at arm's length. Death has become a distant reality to most of us in North America.

It is not this way in many other cultures, nor has it always been this way here. Why is it this way now? I think it is for two reasons. First, our society has become a culture of the "moment." We are encouraged not to live in the past, and we seldom seriously consider the "hereafter" until its inevitability becomes the "here and now."

The second reason is a mixed blessing. Our medical community has so invested itself in life–sickness and death are fought with such zeal–that we now enjoy nothing less than the world's greatest healthcare system. In our methodological high-tech world, death is an opponent. As such, when some doctors lose a patient, as every doctor will, they feel as if they have failed. Death represents failure.

1

Hospice believes that death is not a failure of medicine.

Lost within all our technology is the concept of a natural death. "Quantity" of life has become confused with "quality" of life. Strange though it may seem, when faced with death today, we must sign a legal document to keep from being hooked up to some machine. We must ask permission to be allowed to die naturally, as God intended.

The true failure is that our dying are not being served. And it is precisely for this reason that Dr. Kevorkian has arrived. No one wants to see a loved one die in pain. But because so many are doing so, some have embraced this pathologist and allowed him to do something that we believe God did not intend humankind to do.

Hospice represents a positive alternative. But even with the information superhighway, this news is slow to get out.

"What is hospice?" I asked my father's physician in December of 1994. I had been involved in healthcare for over six years and had never heard of it. At that time, I represented the other side of medicine–the pharmaceuticals I sold were developed to prolong life.

My father was dying. I knew that he was sick, but I had never entertained the idea that he might actually die, that he might leave my mother, my sisters, and me, never to be with us again. I did not know how to act, or even how to feel. But feel I did. I began to ask questions that had not occurred to me before, questions that this book will explore. I look back on that time and wonder how I could have been so unprepared, why the concept was so alien to me. My ignorance intensified the most emotional time of my life.

As my family struggled to come to terms with a reality we had never faced, we soon realized that the hospice team was not there to push us into a program. Simply put, they were there to walk with us through the most difficult time of our lives. They alleviated my father's pain, taught us how to make him comfortable, offered practical advice on legal matters, allowed us to voice our anger and fears without judgment, and prayed with us when we so desired. They could not take away our pain; they could not solve our family squabbles. They just helped.

An enduring memory is of Henrietta, the hospice nurse, sitting at the end of my father's bed as he left us, unobtrusive, her head bowed as she prayed. You see, hospice helped us to understand and accept that this moment was his time to go. My father died encircled by those he loved, and he died held by those who loved him. And he deserved, as we all do, to leave this world in such a way. It was at once the most painful experience of my life and the most profound. I have thanked God every day since that I was there with my family.

Dame Cicely Saunders, the architect of the modern hospice movement, says, "What I do is allow patients to speak for themselves and to suggest that what we ought to do is to give them safe conduct."

No one is suggesting that death is easy or that it was meant to be easy. It very obviously is not, and for that reason, hospice represents a difficult choice. This is the challenge we face today–because of its intimate association with death, many people view the concept of hospice as too depressing. The result is that many are not being reached and served.

The questions we should ask are: Why do so many of us find ourselves so unprepared for death and so fearful of it? Why is hospice such a unique idea in healthcare today? Dr. Tim Siler, a friend and hospice physician, once said to me, "It's ironic that, as a society, we can passionately debate the merits of physician-assisted suicide and yet, within our own families, be so uncomfortable discussing our own mortality."

Like many experiences in our lives, death is really all in how we look at it. It sounds simple enough, I know, but death in our culture is anything but simple, as the stories herein will show. It is our inclination to avoid that which we fear and yet, when we face our fears, what do we learn about ourselves? We can hold death at arm's length or we can embrace it. Death is a sacred journey, whether we learn this in this life or the next. And hospice can be a labor of the love of many in making that journey.

It has been my honor to assist this earnest group of women with their book about hospice. Educating people about hospice has also been my vocation for over two years now. I have learned, as have Denise, Cindy, Shelly, Ann, and Bobbie, that the mission of hospice is, perhaps, more about life than it is about death.

---

[1]Kahil Gibran, *The Prophet* (New York: Alfred A. Knopf, 1971), p. 80.

Chapter One

Death and Dying

Denise Glavan

*Now a certain man was ill, Lazarus of Bethany,
the village of Mary and her sister Martha. Mary
was the one who anointed the Lord with
perfume and wiped his feet with her hair; her
brother Lazarus was ill. So the sisters sent a
message to Jesus, "Lord, he whom you love is
ill"…*

*When Mary came where Jesus was and saw
him, she knelt at his feet and said to him,
"Lord, if you had been here, my brother would
not have died." When Jesus saw her weeping,
and the Jews who came with her were also
weeping, he was greatly disturbed in spirit and
deeply moved…Jesus began to weep.*

John 11:1–3, 32–33, 35

As John said in his introduction, death is a subject most of us are all too happy to avoid. And why wouldn't we? None of us wants to face the inevitability of our mortality or that of our loved ones. When death occurs, we experience an array of emotions, none of which are pleasant. For too many of us today, death is a fearful experience, because it is the unknown. And with the unknown come questions.

Is there life after death? If there is, where do we go when we die? What will happen to my family when I am gone?

Consequently, we might deny death or pretend that it will not occur in our lives. But then, of course, death comes. And when it does, we find that we do not understand it and are unprepared to deal with it. How can we equip ourselves, so that we may have the knowledge and understanding to deal with this thing called death?

David was my 17-year-old brother. In 1988, he died in a car wreck. Driving home from work late one evening, he rounded a corner at a speed estimated to be close to 80 miles per hour. This was in a residential area where the speed limit was 35 miles per hour.

He lost control of his car which swerved into a curb. It slammed into the opposite curb so violently that it broke the back wheel off. The car then flew into the air, flipped over, and crashed into a house. My brother was catapulted from his car and killed.

We will never know exactly why he was driving so fast. He was young, and like the young, he lived life to the fullest. On his route home, this particular curve in the road probably tempted him often. We have speculated that, more than likely, he continuously "pushed the outside of the envelope" around this curve in his car. And because of that, he died.

I was 33 years old. I had never experienced the loss of one so close to me before. I had never experienced this thing called death at all. I could not believe that this was happening. Death happened to other people, not to my family and me.

Later, at my parents' home, a minister came to pay his respects. As we walked into the dining room, he said to me, "My brother died in a car wreck too. He gave me the gift of death. Your brother has given you the same gift."

I thought, *What? How can you say this to me? If this is a gift, I don't want it! I don't want to hear this.* All I could think was, *I've lost my precious brother.* His death changed me forever. I began to read every book I could find on the subject. It forced me to ask questions, to try to uncover some meaning in it all, but mostly to find an answer to the one question, *Why?* My questions eventually led me to hospice.

———

I met Betty in June of 1994. At the time, I served as Director of Chaplains at a hospice in Oklahoma City. Betty was 68 years old and dying of lung cancer. When I first walked in, she was sitting at the kitchen table smoking a cigarette. Her oxygen tank was turned off and her nosepiece was pushed up on her forehead. Though a confirmed smoker, she understood the dangers of smoking around oxygen.

"Hello. Who are you?" she asked. We began to talk. During our conversation, she pulled out another cigarette and asked, "Do you mind if I smoke?"

"No," I replied.

But she must have read something in my expression because she asked, "Why should I quit now, Denise? It's too late. I'm dying. Why should I quit one of the few things that still gives me pleasure?"

So began my relationship with this feisty woman. The next time I saw Betty, she had just returned home from a weekend trip. She had celebrated the Fourth of July with her family, and it had been the best time she had had in a very long while. She had even slept out under the stars. Betty so loved her family and life. She was less feisty this time, more reflective of her condition. It was with a sad smile that she told me, "I doubt that I will see another Fourth."

Betty's final wish, her primary goal, was to attend her granddaughter's wedding on August 7. But the wedding was to be held out of state, and she worried that she might not be healthy enough to go. Still, every time I visited, she would show me all the different things she had bought for her granddaughter. And she would show me what new thing she had bought for herself. She was so excited!

On the Wednesday before the wedding, Betty suffered a multitude of seizures and fell into a coma. Her daughter called me. When I arrived that day, the entire family was crying. They had decided they could not leave their "Momma." The rest of the party, they agreed, would just have to get along without them.

This was especially frustrating because Betty's family was to be actively involved in the wedding. They were to provide the wedding cake and decorations. As I counseled with them, I reminded them how much their mother wanted to go to this wedding and how important it was to her.

"Do you feel that she would really want *all* of you to stay here with her? Do you think she would want you to miss the wedding?" I asked them.

Tearfully, the family decided that some would go and some would stay. I said a prayer with them and left as they made final arrangements. Then I went in and sat down beside Betty. For a while, I just watched her peaceful face. And I thought, *You're such a wonderful woman. How much you have blessed my life.*

Then I began to speak to her, even though I knew she could not respond.

"God loves you, Betty. He knows how much you want to go to your granddaughter's wedding. But sometimes, things don't quite work out as we had hoped. Part of your family is going to go to the wedding for you, as you would want them to. But some of them want to stay and be with you."

I had no way of knowing whether she heard me or not. I hoped she had. I said one more prayer and left.

As I drove home, I was overcome with sadness. *She will not be able to go to her granddaughter's wedding,* I thought. *She will not realize her final wish.*

Not more than fifteen minutes later, I received a page. I called back immediately. "Denise!" Betty's daughter shouted into the phone. "No sooner had you walked out of the house than mother sat upright in her bed! She said, 'Well, I'm ready! Let's go to the wedding!'" Now overcome with happiness, I tried to blink back my tears. The very next day, the family left for the wedding.

I was anxious to see her after she returned. As we sat and talked, she excitedly described the wedding.

"Denise, I walked down that aisle with a grandson on each arm. I made it! Thanks to God, you, and hospice."

Her daughter then said, "You should have seen her with her head held high."

Lung cancer frequently metastasizes (spreads) to the brain. As this happens, it becomes increasingly difficult for a person to hold his or her head up for any length of time. Betty's condition had progressed to this extent.

"It was a miracle!" her daughter said. "Only days before, she could walk only with the assistance of her walker." All Betty wanted was to attend the ceremony. That she could do so, head proudly held high, was indeed a miracle.

Ten days later, Betty died. Were it not for hospice, Betty would very probably have spent her final days in a hospital. More than likely, she would not have gone to her granddaughter's wedding. Hospice gave Betty the opportunity to *live and die* at home–with dignity, love, care, and support.

———

In his book *The Hospice Movement,* Sandol Stoddard writes, "The Latin word, *hospice,* means both host and guest. This, in itself, is interesting, since it puts the spotlight on a process, an interaction between human beings, that was once perceived as simple and mutual."[1]

But what was once perceived as simple and common is now an experience that is alien to us. Webster's defines hospice first as a shelter for travelers and second as a homelike facility for the care of the terminally ill. Today, hospice has evolved into a concept of care.

Hospice care can be delivered in private homes, nursing homes, and, on rare occasions, hospitals. Some states have in-patient hospices. These are facilities provided just for terminally ill patients. They are homelike places where patients will reside until they die.

Ideally, hospice offers the option to remain at home, in an environment where the patient feels safe and comfortable, away from the sterile confines of a hospital. Hospice tries to establish a setting that gives the terminally ill dignity, privacy, and some measure of control over the remainder of their lives.

Stoddard writes, "It is our attitude toward death, I believe, that has so badly skewed and spoiled our contemporary sense of how persons who are well ought to relate to persons who are sick. In America...death is un-American."[2]

Further complicating matters is the attitude of our medical culture. Arnold Tony once remarked, "The death of a patient is perceived as a humiliation and an outrage by the average physician in our culture; to the nursing staff in an acute care hospital, it feels like a personal defeat."

Hospice does not look upon death as a defeat. Hospice gives "hope in a hopeless situation." It encourages the terminally ill and their families to come to terms with death. It helps them say good-bye to each other. Hospice's hope is to establish an atmosphere in which the patient and family can positively deal with their fears and concerns.

Not all terminal patients are appropriate for hospice. Being "hospice-appropriate" means that a patient understands that he or she is dying, and after being fully informed of all options, *chooses* palliative, or comfort, measures only. There are those who will seek aggressive treatment for their disease until their last dying breath. Hospice understands this and does not try to recruit them. This is their choice; it is their life. We only hope that these patients are informed of their options.

Ellen, a woman I knew long before I became involved with hospice, was dying. She was afraid to die. She did not believe in God and was terrified of what might happen after she died. As her time drew near, she demanded that the nurse stay with her. Just before she died, she looked desperately at the nurse and said, "Do whatever it takes, but don't you dare let me die!"

Ellen was never made aware of the option of hospice. If she had been, things might have been very different for her.

In our society, we strive to maintain our youth. Life is for the living! In advertisements, we might hear, "Create the body you wish to have! Call today for a free consultation!" We encourage the mentality that youthfulness is all-important, while the not-so-subtle message is that old age and death are to be avoided at all costs.

When we find that we have a terminal illness, like Ellen, we beg to be saved–no matter what, no matter the cost. And when our doctors cannot save us, even when death is inevitable, we lash out in fear and anger. With our emphasis on youth and perfection, we have set ourselves up for failure.

We have lost sight of the fact that death is a part of life. It is going to happen. At some point, we are going to die. No one is exempt. All we can do, even with our technology, is postpone death for a while and try to improve the quality of life we have remaining.

Hospice deals with this stigma of death daily. It is our ongoing dilemma that so many are unprepared for death. We have a right to die with dignity, surrounded by those we love. We have a right to compassionate care. We have a right to die free of guilt. We have a right to have some measure of control over our final days. Hospice strives to create this environment.

Those who work in hospice are frustrated that so many wait until they have days, perhaps hours, left to live before they seek our services. Even when this happens, we can help, but too often, all we can really offer is crisis management. We cannot adequately perform the mission of hospice.

We understand that if you, or someone you love, were told that you had only six months to live, it would frighten you. Why wouldn't it? Who wants to admit that they are close to death? And so one of our first reactions is anger, anger that we are even sick at all.

Sandol Stoddard writes further, "We have begun to realize, I believe, that the enemy all along was not death, but our own unwillingness to incorporate its reality into our consciousness."[3] So we avoid hospice as if it were a plague, as if *it* were the problem.

The Hospice Medicare Benefit serves those with a life expectancy of six months or less. This does not mean that a terminally ill person *will* die in six months, only that, given the natural progression of the disease, death might occur in that time frame. Of course, only God knows exactly when the moment of death will come. Hospice gives us the blessed opportunity to be a part of someone's life…and death. As Stoddard so eloquently writes, "Death is a hospitable act."[4]

Hospice is true holistic care. We are a team of physicians, nurses, home health aides, social workers, chaplains, bereavement counselors, and volunteers all ministering to the physical, emotional, and spiritual well-being of the terminally ill person and his or her family. Hospice nurses are on call twenty-four hours a day. The social worker, chaplain, and volunteer visit on a regular basis, if so desired.

Hospice tries to establish an atmosphere of love and support for the family and friends as they walk this "sacred journey." Sometimes, this team *becomes* the family, so that the dying will not be alone.

Norman Vincent Peale shares a beautiful story about life and death:

> Now, if a baby still within his mother's womb could talk, he might say, "This is a wonderful place. It's warm. I'm fed. I'm taken care of. I like it here." And if someone said to him, "But you cannot stay here. You must move on. You're going to die out of this place, for you are going to another world." That baby would then look upon the process of birth as if it were death, since it would be the end of the world he knew.
>
> But look what happens now! He is cradled in loving arms. Everybody loves him, and he comes to love this world too. It's even better than the one in which he once had been. He learns to crawl, walk, run, laugh and play. He grows. He marries and has a family. And he grows older. One day he is told, "You're going to die." He protests, "I love this world.

I love my wife and children. I don't want to die."
But he does die to this world, and then he is born
into the next.

And look what happens! Once again, there are
loving faces to greet him. He is surrounded by mu-
sic sweeter than he has ever heard. He cannot believe this new world for it is even better than the one
he had left. And he says, "Why was I so afraid of this
thing called death, when, as I now know, it is really
life instead?"[5]

Why was I so afraid of this thing called death?

I was afraid because, for me, it was a dark, unknown
thing, something with which I had no experience. And I
had made no attempt to face it in my life until it faced me.
Death took my brother and did not afford me the opportunity to say good-bye. For that reason, I will always wish to
see his smile, to touch his hand, and to hear his laughter
once again.

As you read this book, you will look at death...and life.
These two certainties go hand in hand–death is a part of
life. Hospice can give hope in a time where there is none.
Hospice walks with the terminally ill and their families
throughout this sacred journey.

It is our hope that the strategies and methods described
here will equip you to deal with death and its many issues
along the way, into the here...and after.

---

[1]Sandol Stoddard, *The Hospice Movement* (New York: Vintage Books, 1992),
p. 4.

[2]Ibid., p. 6.
[3]Ibid., p. 8.
[4]Ibid., p. 7.
[5]Norman Vincent Peale; source untraced.

CHAPTER TWO

Was It Ethical? Was It Legal? Bobby's Story

Cindy Longanacre

*Nature's first green is gold, her hardest
        hue to hold.
Her early leaf's a flower; but only so an hour.
Then leaf subsides to leaf. So Eden
        sank to grief,
So dawn goes down to day. Nothing
        gold can stay.*

Robert Frost[1]

Bobby was a 41-year-old man, husband and father of two. His wife Pam was loving, loyal, and devoted to her husband. Together they struggled to beat the cancer that had invaded his body and disrupted their lives. As an oncology nurse at the hospital where Bobby received his chemotherapy, I had tended to him. After many months, it became clear that Bobby was losing the battle.

Each time he entered the hospital, he had lost more weight and was weaker than the time before. Instead of coming for treatment only, he began to be hospitalized due to complications of his disease and also for the side effects of his chemotherapy.

On what was to be Bobby's last admission to the hospital, I recognized with a single glance that he would soon leave us. He could barely walk. His skin was stretched taught across his tall frame. His blood counts were so low that we immediately began transfusions. And yet a fierce determination to live shone from his sunken eyes. He continually referred to the time when he would be well and could return to his job. He saw these latest signs of decline as temporary setbacks that angered him but would soon be overcome.

As I listened to him, I tried to remain neutral in the face of his frustration and rage. I could clearly see what Bobby did not want to admit–he was dying. I suspected that Pam could see this as well. Because I knew that a person could not be forced into acceptance, I wanted to provide Bobby support, while at the same time not engendering false hope. I also wanted to give him some sense of control over his situation.

Time was getting short. There was a distinct possibility that Bobby's heart or lungs could fail at any moment. It was time to talk about a DNR, a do not resuscitate order.

A DNR means that if a person's heart or lungs stop functioning, nothing will be done to restart them. Resuscitation was developed for patients who need assistance to overcome a medical crisis but who still have a chance to recover. With progressive conditions such as Bobby's lung cancer, even if we were able to get his heart and lungs going again, there was no possibility of a cure. *We would be bringing him back only to let him die again.* Instead of giving Bobby a fighting chance of recovery, we would merely be prolonging his death.

The day after Bobby's admission to the hospital, I found Pam alone in the family room. I gently explained to her that I had several concerns. Bobby's condition was very serious, and it was possible he could go into cardiac or respiratory arrest. We needed to talk about that situation so that, were this to occur, we would know how to proceed. It was important that Bobby's wishes be known and honored.

Unfortunately, Bobby's physician was not comfortable with this type of conversation. He had not discussed with them that Bobby had now reached the terminal stages of his disease. He had not discussed Bobby's wishes in regard to resuscitation or even the option of palliative care. On the other hand, this physician did not object when nurses broached these topics and almost always agreed to the requested changes in the focus of treatment.

I had the feeling that while Pam was surprised by what I was telling her, she was not totally shocked. Obviously numb from my statements, she still asked several questions. She then thanked me for talking with her so openly, shed a few tears, and said she would think about what I had told her. She would talk with me later. Straightening her shoulders, she went back to Bobby.

By late morning, she sought me out to say that she was ready to approach Bobby about a DNR, and she wanted to do so that afternoon when the physician made his daily rounds. When the doctor arrived, I filled him in on my conversations with Pam. While he agreed to discuss the subject, his reluctance was apparent. He was never comfortable discussing a patient's mortality. By not being able to keep his patients alive, he believed he had failed them. To even suggest that they consent to a DNR, he felt he was destroying what little hope remained.

Seeing his hesitance, I feared he would make no mention of the larger issues of Bobby's overall condition or the option of changing the focus of his treatment to palliative care rather than aggressive measures. I could only hope that the topic of a DNR would open the door for a broader discussion.

It is the physician's responsibility to inform his or her patient about the patient's condition and all of the options for treatment. But when the prognosis is poor, physicians are often disinclined to do so. It is the nurse's responsibility to be at the bedside. And it is the nurses who have to watch the patient struggle with the consequences of these decisions.

Standing at Bobby's bedside, the physician asked general questions about how he was feeling. As was his habit, he then began edging toward the doorway of Bobby's room, as if to leave. I quickly said, "Bobby, we need to talk with you about something else. Your condition is very serious. It is possible that your heart or lungs could stop working. We need to know how you would want us to react in that situation."

Bobby looked at me and asked, "What are you trying to say?"

This was a perfect opportunity for the doctor to address Bobby's terminal state. I glanced at him, trying to signal this. He simply looked at the chart in his hand and waited for me to respond.

"We are required to assume that you would want full resuscitation if you go into cardiac or respiratory arrest. I am not sure that's what you want. If you don't, we must have a do-not-resuscitate order on the chart before we can honor that wish."

Suddenly, Bobby became angry and visibly agitated. He spoke with great hostility in his voice when he said, "I can't believe you are saying this to me! Of course I want everything done! I have a wife and two kids who are counting on me! If you people are giving up on me, I'll find someone who is ready to help me live! I don't even want to talk about this—now or ever!"

In the face of his reaction, the physician quickly left the room. Bobby's response had only reinforced this doctor's conviction. I remained long enough to assure Bobby that my concern was only that his wishes be fulfilled and that he be given the opportunity to make an informed choice. One glance at Pam's stricken face told me that she felt the same as I—the choice that Bobby was making was *not* an informed one.

The doctor had not been open and honest with Bobby about the gravity of his condition and the futility of a resuscitative effort. The conversation should have begun with a discussion of Bobby's poor response to treatment and his overall decline. We could then have discussed what resuscitation meant and the probable outcome in this case. None of this happened. We had only succeeded in alienating our patient.

By the time I returned to the nurses' station, the physician had left. I was seething inside. I told myself I should have known better than to expect this doctor to handle the conversation appropriately. I mulled it over and over in my mind, thinking of how I should have approached it. Mostly I thought, *We have very little time, and Bobby is too angry to talk to us anytime soon. We blew it.*

Bobby remained sullen all day and spoke to me only in monosyllables. I feared that the close, trusting relationship we had developed had suffered irreparable damage. I spoke to Pam alone again before the end of my shift. She confirmed that she, too, was appalled at how the situation was handled and at Bobby's response to it. She began to cry and said, "What are we going to do? I know he's dying." I gave her a hug and assured her that I would be back the following day; we would work through this together.

When I returned the next morning, the night nurse pulled me aside. "Cindy, I need to tell you something…Bobby died last night."

My first response was one of disbelief. I felt my face go pale and tears welled in my eyes. I could only think, *No! Not yet. We aren't ready!*

"Karen," I said, "that isn't funny."

She saw my reaction, hugged me, and said, "I wouldn't joke about something like that. I'm so sorry. Pam decided when he arrested that she didn't want anything done. We didn't call a code. She said to thank you for your help."

I spent a few minutes in the restroom pulling myself together. I had many other patients who needed me. I would do my grieving later. I was also going to have to work through my anger with the physician who could not bring himself to talk to his patient.

That afternoon, I was charting outside a patient's room when I felt a hand touch my arm. I looked up and saw Pam standing there. We embraced each other and immediately began to cry.

"Pam, I'm so sorry," I said as I wept. "I wanted to be here for you when it happened."

She pulled back, shook me slightly, and said, "You *were* with me—in spirit. I want you to know how very hard it was for me to drive sixty miles and walk back into this hospital. But I *had* to come back to thank you. If you had not talked with me yesterday, I would not have been prepared to make the decision for Bobby when the time came. We obviously would never have heard it from that doctor. I know Bobby said he wanted to be resuscitated, but I loved him too much to do that to him. I can't thank you enough for being honest with me. It made all the difference in the world."

———————

Patients always deserve to hear the truth. It is a right that should not be censored or infringed upon in any way. How can we expect people to make good decisions if they do not have all the information they need? We do not take away hope when we give counsel based on our knowledge and experience.

When our professional training and clinical judgment tell us a patient is dying, it is still possible we could be wrong. Medicine is an inexact science and miracles happen every day. And yet, if we do not relay the facts as we see them, we extend *false hope*. Some believe that false hope is better than no hope at all. I disagree. I believe that there is always hope, albeit in different forms. Even when someone is facing death, there is still hope: hope for a peaceful, pain-free experience, hope for the opportunity to make amends or to say goodbye. These are valid goals to work for.

Honesty is the basis for acting legally and ethically in issues surrounding death and dying. Without honesty, we are denying people the right to make their own choices. This is an ethical principle known as "autonomy." It is considered to be the most important ethical principle in healthcare, even above the preservation of human life.

It is also a right. Everyone has the right to refuse medical treatment at any time, *even if that decision results in harm to them.* Our role as healthcare providers includes being a "patient advocate," one who ensures that patients understand the choices they have and then honor and support whatever choice they make. Is it not ironic that we should need such an advocate in the first place?

Our healthcare system is designed so that all patients will have everything possible done to *extend* their lives, unless they specify otherwise. This is probably the best approach. We should all have access to the very best care that will give us the chance of survival and recovery. But when recovery is not possible, or even likely, such as in Bobby's case, and we do not wish to have life-extending treatment, we must take legal steps to ensure that our wishes are fulfilled.

While Bobby had stated that he did wish to be resuscitated, he was not making an informed choice. "Informed consent" is defined as the following: First, a person must have decision-making capacity; then, the patient must have all information about treatment that a reasonable person would need to make a decision. The patient must be able to comprehend the information and must know about treatment alternatives and the risks and benefits of all treatment options. Finally, the patient must know the implications of refusing all treatment and be able to act without coercion.

Other than having decision-making capacity, Bobby met none of these criteria when he stated that he wanted resuscitation. Because of the doctor's reluctance and the fact that the situation escalated so quickly, Bobby was not given the information he needed to make an informed decision. Pam's choice to forego the "code" (resuscitation efforts) met more of the conditions for informed consent because of my conversations with her. She understood the true situation and, therefore, her wishes were honored.

Obviously, this was not an ideal situation. Had the doctor been honest with Bobby much earlier, we could have obtained informed consent for either a DNR or a full-code status (full resuscitative efforts, including CPR and a ventilator) from Bobby himself. In Oklahoma, Pam had no real legal grounds to make this choice for Bobby. But at the time of this incident, it was standard practice to follow the family's wishes when a patient became incapacitated, even if those wishes differed from the patient's.

Perhaps what took place was not technically legal, but I will always believe that it was more ethical than allowing a futile code that would possibly have prolonged Bobby's suffering and *death.*

In 1992, the Patient Self-Determination Act was passed. This federal law allows us to make choices in advance about potential crisis medical situations, such as if we are terminally ill or in an irreversible coma. The idea was to preserve patients' autonomy, even after they became unable to make their own choices (incapacitated). It also allows for the appointment of a third party (a healthcare proxy) to make medical decisions for the incapacitated person. The actual format of the document and restrictions placed upon it vary somewhat from state to state.

Everyone over the age of eighteen should have such a document. We never know when a tragic event will occur, one that will leave us unable to communicate to our loved ones and healthcare providers exactly what we would want done. An Advance Directive is a legal document that is our best assurance of making our wishes known and honored.

It is not enough to simply fill out the form, however. We need to discuss with our family and physician what we have decided and *why.* In order to make choices for us, they must understand something of our values and beliefs. There are too many different scenarios to be provided for in a single document. Interpretation is often required, but this cannot accurately be done without knowing beforehand what an individual considers quality of life to be. Each person's idea of quality of life is unique and distinct from another's. It is not an easy thing to second-guess.

In matters of life and death, legal and ethical concerns will almost always arise. In order for the terminally ill person's death to occur as he or she desires, certain preparations should be made. Keep in mind that these preparations are subject to local laws, which can vary widely from state to state. Before completing these arrangements, check with your hospice team, physician, or attorney. They can advise you on the options available in your area.

While the ending to Bobby's story was not what I would have wished, I was still able to make a difference for Pam. Sometimes we face a paradox in healthcare: What is legal is not always necessarily ethical, and what is ethical is not always necessarily legal.

Maybe we should ask ourselves, Why?

---

[1]Robert Frost, *The Poetry of Robert Frost* (New York: Holt, Rinehart and Winston, 1969), p. 222.

CHAPTER THREE

Hope in the Midst of Suffering

Denise Glavan

Precious in the sight of the LORD
is the death of his faithful ones.

Psalm 116:15

I cry out for help,
Where are you God?
I pull my hair and shake
my fists and ask, why?
I get down on my hands and knees
asking for strength,
courage,
and guidance.
Then I sit in the silence of the early dawn,
all alone.
All by myself.
Praying for help and understanding.
Praying and praying.

> Can you hear me, Lord?
> Can you hear me?
> Are You there?
> Do You care?
> Where are You, Lord?
> I need You now, Oh, how I need You.
>
> Denise

Have you ever felt like that? You probably have at one time or other. There is a name for this feeling. Lloyd John Ogilvie, in his book titled *Ask Him Anything,* calls it "the night of suffering."[1] It is a time of anguish when we cry out for help, and it can occur when we least expect it, day or night.

April 19, 1995. I served as the director of chaplaincy at a hospice in Oklahoma City, and on that morning, I was in a meeting in an upstairs conference room. At 9:02 a.m., a shock wave jarred our building seconds before a heavy, resounding *BOOM!* Bewildered, we looked at each other and asked, "What was *that?*"

We ran downstairs, yelling for everyone to evacuate the building. Outside, at first, we could not see the source of the explosion. Shortly, a black Mercedes screeched to a halt beside us and the driver shouted, "A building downtown just blew up!"

Thirteen miles due south, the north side of the Murrah Federal Building had just been blasted into ruins, and 168 men, women, children, and babies lay dead or dying.

We looked back in that direction and were able to see a billowing cloud of smoke rising in the sky, growing larger by the second. We rushed back inside and turned on the TV. After a few moments of listening to the chaos being reported, I went straight to my boss.

"I know the head of chaplaincy at Presbyterian Hospital. Should I call him?"

"Yes," he said. "Let's see if we can help."

I called my friend Ken Blank, and he said, "By all means! We can use you." I arrived at the hospital at 9:30.

The hospital had hastily set up two areas—a triage next to the ER for the injured and a waiting room in the auditorium for family and those looking for family. I walked immediately to triage.

Initially, all I could do was hold their hands. I held the hand of a woman as the nurses removed pieces of glass from her body. She gripped my hand tightly, as if I were her lifeline.

"Does anyone know what happened?" she asked. At this time, no one did and no one would for hours. "My sister is here somewhere," she told me. "Would you find her and let her know that I'm okay?"

She described her and I walked to the auditorium. As I searched, a man frantically rushed up to me.

"I've lost my wife! I can't find her! I've been to the other hospitals and I can't find her! Oh God, help me! Please, somebody help me!" He embraced me and then began to sob uncontrollably. The poor man was physically and emotionally drained. I held him for a good ten minutes. When he regained control, I asked him if he would rest while I found someone to assist him.

"Yes," he sighed and sat down. We said a quick prayer and I left.

So began the most horrific day of my life. The carnage I witnessed firsthand was something no child of God should ever have to see, and yet, there it was. Never have I felt so needed, and rarely have I felt so helpless. To say that my life was changed forever cannot begin to describe what happened to me or to so many others.

I saw things that I wish I could forget—bodies, parts of bodies; injured of different races, ages, and genders; ragged and bloody clothing; screams of pain and the frightened, imploring eyes of family searching for family.

April 19, 1995, a bright and sunny Oklahoma springtime day, was a blur of confused activity, desperation, and sorrow. As the sunlight faded into a night of frantic heroism,

I found myself at the First Christian Church on 36th and Walker. The families there pleaded for answers to their questions.

"Why is this happening?"

"Why is this happening to *me*?"

"Oh, God help me!"

"She just *has* to be alive."

"Why would anyone do this?"

"Why did God allow this to happen?"

"Why me?"

"Why my mother?"

"Why? This just can't be happening!"

"What am I going to do if she (or he) is dead?"

I met Bobby, a chaplain for the Teamsters, at the First Christian Church Wednesday night. We were drawn together by the catastrophe and soon began to work effectively as a team. Like me, he had worked at the site of the bombing all day.

Later that night, around 11:30, we went back. As we stood amid the rubble and rescue workers, Bobby turned to me and said, "Denise, we're short of chaplains. Can you help us tomorrow morning at the morgue?"

"Of course," I said. There was no way I could not go.

I arrived at 7:30 a.m. Thursday. Throughout the day, I spoke with those charged with identifying the bodies. As the day progressed, so did their anger. I listened as they expressed helplessness and frustration, pain and sorrow. As I prayed over the bodies in the morgue and for the families of the victims, I tried to comprehend the incomprehensible. The world knew now that someone had deliberately and maliciously committed this act.

One memory sticks with me, one that, try as I might, I cannot forget. It comes unbidden. As I prayed over the many bodies that were being brought into the morgue, a man pulled from a plastic bag a little pair of *Lion King* tennis shoes. When I saw those tiny, empty shoes, I thought, *Oh God!* Lion King *tennis shoes? Where is this baby?* As tears rolled down my face, the insanity of that day forced me to look up and silently scream, *WHY?*

Thursday night, I returned to the First Christian Church and the Notification Team began their work. On this night, we notified only two families. We would begin our work in earnest on Friday morning. As the next day dawned, I counseled the others on what to say and how to say it. I also cautioned them about responses they might expect in return.

"Some may faint, some might scream, wail, or curse at you. Some might become angry or violent and strike out at you. Some may blame you," I told them. "Try to understand; in this kind of situation, it's common for people to lash out. You just happen to be there; you are convenient. In whatever manner they choose to express themselves, they are expressing feelings and emotions we can only guess at. *And they are not wrong to express them.* Lastly, never assume it is appropriate to touch someone. Always ask first."

For three straight days, from early morning until midnight, we were the bearers of a harsh and final truth: *Your loved one is dead.*

The memorial service on Sunday afternoon was the culmination of five mind-numbing days. A number of us walked wearily up and down the aisles, checking on families and hoping to be a comforting presence to those we had come to know.

As I walked, a man reached out to me and said joyfully, "Denise! Denise, is that you?" For a moment, I did not recognize him. "Don't you remember me, from Presbyterian Hospital? I'm the man who couldn't find his wife!"

"Oh, yes!" I said and we hugged each other. "It's so good to see you."

"I wanted to thank you…and tell you the rest of the story." I looked into his eyes and he said, "I found my wife! She's here. I want to introduce you to her." I began to cry. This was the only good piece of news I had seen or heard since the bombing. I wept for joy, and I wept in relief. All I could do was weep.

Have you ever observed what happens when you throw a pebble into a pond? The stone causes waves of water to ripple out in ever-widening rings. Long after the stone disappears, the ripples continue to flow outward. I thought of this simple analogy many times after that awful week. The repercussions of the bombing, felt most keenly in Oklahoma City, rippled out across America and the world. But the memory of that horror will forever ripple back.

Ogilvie writes, "We all have one of three things in common: We have known the night of suffering, are in the night right now, or are deeply troubled about someone who is. It is in the dark night of suffering, that we readily cry out in anguish, 'O God, where are you?'"[2]

The bombing, of course, did not allow me an opportunity to perform the mission of hospice, but my expertise in bereavement proved invaluable. Those who lost a loved one in this tragedy endured many "a dark night of suffering."

I would like to tell you what I have found to be true and helpful. Before I do, I would like to share with you my understanding of good and evil in this world.

Let me begin with the story of the fall of Adam and Eve. Adam and Eve ate fruit from the tree of the knowledge of good and evil, and suddenly, they were given knowledge. Whereas before, they knew only the bliss of the garden of Eden, now their knowledge encompassed both the good and the bad of life, and something especially new to them—death.

This is their legacy to us. True knowledge means that we cannot fully appreciate the warmth of happiness and joy until we have known pain and sadness; the light never appears as colorful and bright as when we walk out of the cool darkness. Life seldom has more meaning to us than when someone we love dies. Herein lies some understanding of our anguished questions.

If we selected only those parts of life that suited us, then we would limit the extent of our knowledge, and therefore limit ourselves. We do not wish to experience "the dark night of suffering." But, as M. Scott Peck said, a full life will include pain, sickness, and death, and our only alternative is not to live life fully.[3] I, for one, do not want to limit myself, because knowledge is nothing less than God's gift to us. I want to *live* and make choices.

Sometimes, the choices we make are the source of our suffering. So it was with a patient of mine named Linda. I was on vacation when I received a call from our patient care coordinator.

"Denise, we need your help. We have a patient who is refusing to die. She was a battered woman who shot and killed her husband twenty-eight years ago. We know you can help her. You will know what to say to her."

"But I'm on vacation," I protested. "And it's my son's birthday."

"I'm sorry, Denise. There's no one else."

And so I called and talked to Linda's son. For the past five weeks, Linda had lain near death, but she would not let go.

"Twenty-eight years ago, Mom shot and killed our dad," he explained. "He drank too much and beat her. She has never dealt with what happened. She has never so much as discussed it. I know it's eating her up and has been all these years. Mom's afraid to die because she does not believe that she's worthy to go to heaven."

When I arrived, her son ushered me into her bedroom. I had never seen anything like this before. She looked like a survivor of a Nazi concentration camp. She had dark circles under her sunken eyes and skin like yellow parchment. She appeared to be decaying from the inside out. I sat down at her bedside and began to talk to her.

"Linda," I said softly, "sometimes we are put into situations that we have no control over. Sometimes we are forced to make choices that no one should have to make. Sometimes we do things because we can see no other way out. Your son has told me that you believed that this was the only way you could protect your family."

"Linda," I continued, "God loves you. God forgives you. Can you forgive yourself as God forgives you? Can you accept God's love?" As I talked to her, after a while, she began to relax, and the tension slowly drained from her face.

I talked to her for thirty minutes. Then I spoke with her three children.

"Was she a good mother?"

"Yes, she was," they all agreed.

"Do you support her and believe in her? Do you love her?"

"Oh yes!" they said. "We could not have asked for a better mother!"

"Have you told her this? Have you given her permission to die?"

"No," her son said. "I haven't."

"Neither have we," said her daughters.

"She can hear you," I told them. "Tell her these things, and then tell her it's okay to die."

Each one then went to her and told her how special she was. They told her how much they loved her. And then they gave her permission to die.

"It's okay, Mother," they wept.

We prayed. At 4:00 the next morning, Linda finally let go and died peacefully.

It may seem strange that anyone would need our permission to leave this world. We die when it is our time to die; we cannot stave off death, right? But incredible though it may seem, some people will refuse to begin their new journey until they receive whatever dispensation they need from those they are leaving behind.

It is at times like these that simple but carefully chosen words, or a gentle touch, are *critical,* even *required,* affirmations of love and approval. It may appear to us that our loved one is incapable of feeling our embrace or hearing our words of forgiveness or devotion. Such is not the case.

Meg was a wonderful ninety-five-year-old lady who also did not think she was good enough to get into heaven. She had been raised in the era of fire and brimstone evangelicalism. She had gone to church almost every week of her life. She started teaching Sunday school when she was fourteen years old and continued to teach into her late seventies.

She was the type of person who never met a stranger and would help anyone in need. She loved God and was one of the most spiritual persons I have ever met. But as her illness progressed, her fear increased. One night, at 11:00, she paged me.

"Denise, I'm afraid of dying," she said as I sat with her. "I wonder if I have been good enough. How do I know if I am saved? I'm so afraid. Will you hear my confession of faith?"

"Of course," I said. She made her confession, and I assured her that God did, indeed, love her.

"It feels so good," she sighed. "Yes, I know, God does love me."

Three days later, we talked about her long life and many experiences. But once again, her fears and concerns returned. I answered her questions by using her very own words.

"Meg," I said, "God created you. How could God not love you? Do not doubt God's love. You have been a good and faithful servant. You have done everything that God has asked of you. God loves you and forgives you. You are a very special lady and because of that, God has used you many times to carry out his work here on Earth."

But even for those of strong faith, death is still the great unknown. As the end drew near, she asked feebly once more, "Denise, how do I know that God loves me?"

I rubbed her head softly. And then I began to sing to her.

> *Jesus loves me! This I know,*
> *for the Bible tells me so.*
> *Little ones to Him belong;*
> *they are weak, but he is strong.*
> *Yes, Jesus loves me! Yes, Jesus loves me!*
> *Yes, Jesus loves me! The Bible tells me so.*[4]

And then Meg began to sing. As she did, I sat in awe. Her voice was young and strong, more like that of a woman half her age. Tears welled up in my eyes.

And just at that moment, something happened that I have never forgotten and never will. I felt a presence. I felt His presence. It was like nothing I've ever felt before.

"Jesus loves me! This I know…"

And soon after she sang, she died.

It is very common that questions of faith, questions of good and evil, arise as we are dying. When I think of Meg, I think also of this story. It is the story of two men who had grown up together. They went to grade school, high school, and college together. They were lifelong friends. However, one always seemed to have a smile on his face; he always had a positive outlook on life. The other walked around with a dour expression; he was always quick to point out the negative things in the world.

At the end of their lives, the man who had existed so grimly found himself at his friend's bedside as he lay near death. The dying man smiled at him.

"Even now, my friend, you see the good and bright side of life," he said. "I do not understand."

The dying man grasped his friend's hand weakly. "I always tried to do my best, even when times were bad, so that I would have no regrets. I have always tried to live life to the fullest. Because I have lived my life in such a way, I do not have any regrets. I know that it's okay to die. I have said and done all the things that need to be said and done."

When we face death, we may find ourselves struggling with the price of the human experience—the memory of words we failed to say, the kindness we did not acknowledge, wrongs we have committed, the loved ones we have lost. But I believe that this price is a shared one. Let me explain.

Years ago, I had a vision. It was at once horrifying and heavenly. And though parts of it sickened me, I have always felt privileged to see it. I looked out upon the Earth and saw brilliant light and ominous darkness. The darkness hovered over the light. The light reached upward into the darkness and as it did, it illuminated these scenes:

I saw a little girl in a bedroom, backing toward the bed, saying, "Please Daddy, don't do that. Please."

I saw a woman hit by a man so hard that she flew into a wall, screaming, "Oh God! Help me, please!"

I saw eight people in a convenience store, screaming and begging for their lives, and then mercilessly being shot down.

I could hardly bear to watch, and yet I was compelled to do so. Finally, I turned from the darkness and looked behind me. I beheld an essence I believed to be God. A tear slowly rolled down that magnificent face. I realized then, in a moment of surpassing sadness, that I had been seeing and hearing the same things God sees and hears all the time. And I understood, as I never have before, how much God hurts with us.

Though I see atrocities every day, I had never really considered what it must be like for the Father to see this on such a worldwide scale. I truly believe that God is with us, always, and in all things. God is the one sure thing in this world of daily uncertainty. God will see us through all of our problems. God will never leave us or forsake us. God will even walk with us through the valley of the shadow of death.

Our struggle in life, I believe, is learning to rely on God—to put all of our care in God's hands, to be patient, to let go, and let God—

Even when it seems unfair.
Even when we question.
Even when it hurts.
Even when we have to say goodbye.

---

[1]Lloyd Ogilvie, *Ask Him Anything: God Can Handle Your Hardest Questions* (New York Word: Inc./Guideposts, 1981), p. 36.

[2]Ibid.

[3]M. Scott Peck, *The Road Less Traveled* (New York: Simon & Schuster/Touchstone, 1993), p. 16.

[4]Anna B. Warner, 1860.

CHAPTER FOUR

Going Gently

Cindy Longanacre

*For what is it to die but to stand naked in the
wind and to melt into the sun?
And what is it to cease breathing, but to free the
breath from its restless tides,
that it may rise and expand and seek God
unencumbered?*

Kahlil Gibran[1]

In my experience as a hospice nurse, most families, at
some point, usually ask the same questions. These questions
are so simple and so basic that the fact that they must be
asked at all is truly representative of a phenomenon in our
culture—the almost total denial of our own mortality. Let's
look a little closer at these questions.

The first question is usually, *"How much longer will my
loved one live?"* It is asked for several reasons. The family

may be preparing to let go of their loved one. They want to know the time frame that they have to work with. They may need to make arrangements: arrange time off work, make travel plans, or develop schedules so that family members can rotate caregiving duties.

They may have emotional healing to do. They may need to complete relationships by giving and receiving forgiveness. They may need to say goodbye or say I love you.

They want reassurance. They want an answer to a question no one can answer. They *don't* want their loved one to die, so they ask, "How much longer will she [he] live?"

"What will happen as my loved one dies?" This second question reflects a basic lack of understanding about what is a normal physiological process. As our medical technology has advanced, our emphasis has shifted to prolonging life, whatever the case, whatever the cost. It has become the norm for people to die in institutions, rather than at home. This affords us less opportunity to observe the changes that we can expect to occur as someone dies.

The result is that each generation has become more removed from the reality of death. Now, our society treats this topic as a taboo subject, too "morbid" to discuss. In fact, even healthcare workers caring for dying people gain most of their knowledge of death and dying through experience, not formal training. How ironic that the one universal experience we will all share is the one we are least prepared for!

As a result, when told that we, or someone we love, are terminally ill, we find ourselves at a crisis point. Not only do we not know how to care physically for someone who is so sick, we have no idea how to deal with the emotional and spiritual issues that naturally accompany the dying process. It is my hope that by addressing all of these issues, I can remove some of the mystery and fear surrounding this unknown territory.

Only by arming ourselves with knowledge can we truly be of help to people during this most important time. It is an honor and a privilege for us to be allowed to be involved in such an intimate and private experience. We would do well to never forget this and to attempt a balance between helping and intruding, for this *is* a sacred journey.

The honest and correct answer to these fundamental questions is always, "No one really knows for sure." We can, however, make educated guesses. We make these based on the person's disease, rate of deterioration, their health at the time of admission to hospice, and the presence, or absence, of what we refer to as the "signs and symptoms of impending death."

The unknown is always much scarier than actual fact. To prepare caregivers for expected changes, it is important to review the following signs and symptoms. Be aware of this:

Not all of these changes may occur.
They may occur in any sequence.
They may be exhibited months, weeks, or
hours before death.

In general, body systems begin to slow down, eventually ceasing altogether. While we have a timetable of sorts to begin to look for these signals, the actual experience of dying is as individual as the person. *Everyone dies differently.*

The following is a review of the clues that tell us that the end of a person's life is drawing near. For each sign or symptom, comfort measures are listed: practical tasks that may greatly reduce the unpleasant physical changes that generally accompany the dying process and increase the person's quality of life. They also have the added benefit of guiding caregivers to help in a truly meaningful way.

Caregivers want very much to help but are often unsure of exactly what to do. It is important to remember that the *patient* should remain in control of the situation. They should make every decision possible, even such simple things as what to eat, what to wear, and scheduling of activities.

Withdrawal from Surroundings

As the body weakens, most dying people come to the realization that their time is limited. While many have known this intellectually for some time, emotional acceptance often occurs only a short time before death. Some people never achieve this level of acceptance, believing up until the moment of death that a miracle will occur and they will be spared. For them, gentle compassion and support are particularly important.

We cannot take away people's denial, their coping mechanism. A coping mechanism is the way in which a person deals with a situation. Some are healthy and help the person to learn; others are not as healthy and hold the person in a state of confusion. If we attempt to take this away, they will have no way to cope at all.

It is to be hoped that, if the person is willing, we can teach coping mechanisms other than denial, so that he will be able to accept what is happening to him. If, however, a person is unable to do this, support should always be offered, *without judgment,* because we each deal with death in our own way.

Regardless of their level of acceptance, most people do begin to develop their own rituals of withdrawal. They begin to lose interest in the outside world, paying less attention to newspapers or television. They may begin to limit visits from friends and neighbors as they withdraw into their own family circle.

As time passes, they will eventually withdraw from everything outside their own body and retreat inside. While they may appear to be sleeping, it is very likely that much internal work is actually being done. These people are probably processing their lives, weighing their meaning and value. At this point, communication may cease, because words require too much precious energy.

What you can do

Allow the person to sleep, while taking full advantage of periods of wakefulness. Do not feel compelled to follow the same medication or care schedule that you have in the past. Seek the advice of your physician or nurse to ensure that the person's physical symptoms are adequately treated without overly disturbing the dying person.

Although your loved one may be unable to speak to you, do not hesitate to express how much you love him or her and will miss him or her. Contribute to the process of life review by reminiscing with the dying person and family members–this helps validate the value of the person's life. Continue to touch and speak to the person; it is well established that the senses of hearing and touch are the last to be lost.

Remember that, sometimes, just *being with* the person is more important than *doing for.* The very best help may be the comforting assurance that you are present and that you care. Allow the patient to set the agenda; this is the patient's experience, and control belongs to her or him.

Reduced Desire for Food or Drink

This physiological change is particularly difficult for caregivers to accept. Ensuring that someone is adequately fed and hydrated is an integral part of caring for that person. When they begin to refuse food or drink, caregivers often panic, thinking it is their responsibility to ensure nutrition is taken in.

While caregivers are correct that food is what sustains us, they do not realize that it is perfectly natural to stop eating as the body prepares to die. It takes a tremendous amount of energy to process food. Ever notice how sleepy you are after a heavy meal? Because your blood flow has been shunted to your gastrointestinal system, you have less available energy for other physical demands. As body systems begin to fail, energy that might otherwise have been spent processing food is now reserved to keep vital organs functioning as long as possible.

Sometimes caregivers may try anything to get the person to eat, such as resorting to bribes or instilling guilt. Because the dying person's body cannot process food, nausea and/or vomiting often occur. This contributes to physical discomfort as well as a feeling of frustration for the caregiver and patient alike. Remember, it's okay not to eat.

What you can do

Frequently offer, but do not force, food, drink, and medications. Again, your physician or nurse can best advise which medications are absolutely necessary for comfort. Many of these medicines can be given in ways other than by mouth–sublingually (a concentrated form of the medicine dropped under the tongue), by rectal suppository, or transdermally (absorbed through the skin).

The process of dehydration is often of particular concern to families, who may request that intravenous fluids be given to make the person more comfortable. Recent research, however, strongly suggests that dehydration itself is often a comfort measure. I have found this to be true in my own experience, as well.

Artificial hydration can cause problems such as increased fluid in the body collecting in the lungs or arms and legs; increased urination, resulting in a need for frequent bathroom trips or changing of diapers or linen, and increased gastric secretions, which contribute to nausea.

On the other hand, dehydration *prevents* these problems as well as producing a feeling of euphoria. The only unpleasant side effect consistently reported from dehydrated terminally ill patients is dry mouth. This is easily treated with ice chips, small drops of water placed frequently in the mouth, artificial saliva (available over-the-counter at any drug store), or even small sips of water.

Increasing Fatigue

The dying person will become weaker and weaker as body systems fail. He or she will sleep more and more, withdrawing as discussed earlier. Disorientation becomes common as the importance of marking time diminishes and the person sleeps much of the day and night. He or she seems to be focusing less on this world and more on the next.

The person may speak to or see people who are not there, often those who have died before. The dying person may report dreams of a journey to be taken, of someone coming for him or her soon, or another vision of the impending transition.

What you can do

Offer reassurance by your continued presence. Do not argue with the person by stating, "Why, you couldn't possibly

have seen Aunt Mildred. You know she died years ago!"
Calmly accept the statements and gently explore how the
person feels about what is happening to him or her, if that
seems appropriate. If you are not comfortable discussing this
topic, call the hospice and ask for a team member to help you.

Be reassured that this is very common. In my experience, these dreams or visions comfort most patients. *Do not
confuse them with medication-induced hallucinations.* It is the family that finds the experience distressful.

Loss of Ability to Control Bladder and Bowel

A decrease in urinary function will probably occur, due
to less fluid being taken in and a decreased circulation
through the kidneys. Furthermore, as the person becomes
less responsive, bladder and bowel control may be lost. Altogether, this is very common, and most patients appear to
be unaware when it occurs. Because we are always striving
to maintain the person's dignity, good hygiene now becomes
extremely important.

What you can do

Use absorbent, plastic-backed pads to protect bedding.
Dress the person in clothing that allows easy accessibility.
This avoids prolonging the time needed for bathing and
changing. Diapers may be helpful; adult sizes can be found
in any grocery store or may be provided by the hospice
agency.

Ask the hospice nurse or home health aide to show you
how to bathe the person and change linen while the patient
remains in the bed. Provide for privacy while this personal
care is being done; have no more people present than absolutely necessary, and keep the person as covered as possible. *Dignity should be maintained up to and beyond the moment
of death.*

If the person has not urinated in ten to twelve hours,
report this to the hospice nurse. The nurse may need to make
a visit to assess if the person or family needs, or wants, a
urinary catheter inserted. A catheter can relieve a full bladder caused by blockage and/or make personal care easier
for both patient and caregiver.

If the person already has a catheter and no urine appears in the collection bag for six to eight hours, check for kinks in the catheter tubing. If none is observed, the hospice nurse should be notified. A visit may be made to check for blockage of the catheter tubing, which can be irrigated to remove the obstruction.

Changes in Breathing Patterns

Breaths will become irregular, more shallow, and farther apart. There may be periods of apnea (pauses in the person's breathing lasting ten to thirty seconds). The person may seem to be working very hard to breathe and make a moaning noise when exhaling. Oral secretions may collect in the back of the throat and rattle or gurgle as the person breathes through the mouth.

This is known as the "death rattle." It is much more distressful for families than the dying person, who usually appears unaware of it. *It is a very normal phenomenon.* The death rattle is a signal that death is drawing very near. Secretions may dry and become encrusted in the mouth and on the lips.

What you can do

Turning the person on his or her side may help secretions drain instead of pooling in the back of the throat. Thorough, frequent mouth care using oral sponges (a small sponge on a stick, impregnated with mild cleanser) can relieve dry mouth and remove dried secretions. If the person appears to be in distress from excess mucus or shortness of breath, call the hospice nurse, who may assess the need for oxygen, suction, or other treatment.

Changes in Skin

As the person weakens and takes in less nutrition, the skin becomes much more pale. If liver disease is involved, a yellow or even orange tone may be seen in the skin. Elderly patients and those who have been ill for an extended time have very fragile skin that is prone to developing bedsores.

As the person is "actively dying" (hours from death, with body systems rapidly failing), mottling (purplish blotches on the skin) becomes apparent, especially in the arms and legs. The lips and nails may turn a bluish hue. This is caused from lack of proper blood circulation as the heart fails.

What you can do

Good hygiene is very important to prevent bedsores. The hospice may arrange for a special thick pad for the bed, such as a Geo-mat or air pressure mattress, to alleviate pressure and keep bedsores from forming. Once the person ceases moving around in the bed on his own, make sure to change his position at least every two hours.

The hospice nurse can show you how to position the person with pillows to provide the most comfort and prevent pressure areas. Touch and massage can be helpful in stimulating circulation to the skin. Be sure to always ask permission from the person before using this, as it may cause pain or be unacceptable to her.

Control of Pain

Many patients have told me that they do not fear death; it is the pain associated with dying that frightens them. They have envisioned a long, tortured process filled with physical agony and indignities to a body already ravaged by disease. With the proper care, this should never be the case.

All patients have the right to have their pain controlled. With a few isolated exceptions, every patient should have sufficient pain management such that pain does not limit his life's activities. We have the technology and the tools available to us. It is up to us to use them. Because we have no test that will reveal if a person is truly experiencing pain, *we must always believe the person when he reports pain.*

What you can do

Believe the person when she says she hurts. Promptly report any changes in the patient's condition, whether related to pain or some other problem. Often, small problems can be prevented from turning into a major discomfort that is difficult to control. When in doubt, call the hospice nurse. He is your best guide and will always appreciate being kept informed.

If you feel that the dying person is uncomfortable, contact the healthcare workers helping the person. Insist that they continue to try new methods until goals in controlling pain are met. Remember that medications should only be given by licensed healthcare professionals or family members trained in medication administration. If you are a volunteer providing respite for the family, and the person needs medication, call the hospice.

Sometimes people have fears about giving pain medication, particularly narcotics like morphine. They are afraid the person may become addicted. Or they are afraid that if morphine is used "too soon" in the disease, it will stop working and the person will be left in even more excruciating pain. These common concerns are completely unfounded.

Many studies have shown that patients who use narcotics for pain control seldom become addicted to them—statistically, less than 1 percent. Physical dependence will most likely occur, but this is not the same as addiction. Physical dependence results when a person takes a medication routinely over time so that the body becomes adjusted to the presence of the medicine. When the medicine is suddenly stopped, the person experiences withdrawal symptoms. The presence of withdrawal symptoms is not proof that the person is addicted.

If a patient no longer requires the medication, he should be weaned from it, gradually decreasing the dose over a period of time. Physical dependence does occur in cases of addiction, but they are not the same. Addiction is defined as a psychological craving for the euphoric effect of the drug, combined with drug-seeking behavior. People who take narcotics for this euphoric effect (to get "high") are at risk for addiction. This is seldom the case for those who are simply seeking to relieve their pain.

The second fear is not having a strong enough medication for the final stages of illness unless we "save the morphine until we really need it." This fear also has no basis in fact. Morphine is a very effective drug for moderate to severe pain. It has the additional benefit of having no restriction to the dosage that can be used. This means that we can simply increase the amount of medication the person is taking until the pain is relieved.

As long as this is done gradually and appropriately, there is little risk involved. Therefore, there is no reason to wait until the very last weeks or days of a person's life to use morphine for pain control. There are many moral and ethical reasons to use it as early as needed!

When Death Occurs

The death of a hospice patient is obviously not an unexpected event. You and your hospice team have worked together to achieve the goal of a peaceful transition.

If you sense that your loved one is near death, call the hospice nurse. If you need or desire support or assistance, someone will be with you.

Nothing else needs to be done.

Some families prefer to be left alone at this time. This is a very private and intimate moment, and the presence of anyone outside of family is an intrusion. The hospice team will take their cues from you, providing as much or as little support as each family desires.

Most people in *our* society today have never been present at a person's death. The signs of death are:

- No breathing
- No heartbeat
- No response
- Eyes slightly open, no blinking, a fixed stare
- Possible release of bladder and bowel contents
- Jaw relaxed and slightly open

The hospice nurse will come as quickly as possible to verify death. The nurse will make the necessary official calls, including those to the physician and funeral home.

It is hoped that this information has relieved your mind as well as your heart. Having some idea of what to expect, and what to do, can make all the difference. Of course, no one can predict exactly what will occur as someone dies. In my experience, most families' greatest fears are unfounded.

With the assistance of hospice, most patients are able to achieve their goal of a "good death," bringing a measure of peace to their family.

[1]Kahil Gibran, *The Prophet* (New York: Alfred A. Knopf, 1971), p. 81.

CHAPTER FIVE

Maintaining Boundaries

Cindy Longanacre

See first that you yourself deserve to be a giver,
And an instrument of giving.

For in truth it is life that gives unto life—
while you,
Who deem yourself a giver, are but a witness.

Kahlil Gibran[1]

Why do you find yourself reading this book? At this point, you are on the fifth chapter, so we can assume that you are truly interested. Why? Everyone knows that death is a topic we do not talk about, to say nothing of spending hours reading this book!

The answer depends upon your situation. This book was written not only for caregivers who have no personal relationship with the person who is dying (such as professionals and volunteers), but also for those who may be caring for a terminally ill loved one in their family.

While these are two very different perspectives that require unique coping strategies, *boundary setting* must occur in both situations. Otherwise, the caregiver, professional or layperson, may be overwhelmed and unable to do the work. To fully understand how this occurs, let's examine both situations separately.

The Caring Professional or Volunteer

If you are a professional caregiver, your motivation may be personal growth—wanting to learn more about what death will be like when you inevitably experience it. While personal growth will almost certainly happen once you begin the difficult work of coming to terms with mortality, whether yours or someone else's, my guess is that your primary motivation is a desire to help.

You want to feel more comfortable if you have the opportunity to assist someone who is dying. You do not want to feel helpless and afraid in this most human of situations. You want to make a difference in the quality of this experience, whether for yourself or someone you care for.

What motivates you to pick up this book and make the effort to read it is the very quality that will make you an exceptional helper to dying patients and families—you *care*. And yet, helping is an extraordinarily demanding activity that does not always come naturally or easily.

When you commit to caring, you run the risk of compassion fatigue—otherwise known as "burnout." Caring for others with passion and enthusiasm can lead to self-fulfillment, but a bright flame by its very nature is more likely to burn out.

Burnout has three central characteristics: emotional exhaustion, diminished caring, and a strong sense of not being able to do the work any longer. Burnout can make you feel that you have no energy to deal with a single patient, let alone many patients.

A loss of enthusiasm for your work can make you feel helpless. You may doubt your abilities and wonder if what you are doing is really making a difference. This experience can take a tremendous toll on you emotionally and physically.

In fact, it is often true that the most idealistic and committed helpers are the first to experience compassion fatigue. As a helper, *you must maintain a delicate balance between emotional commitment and using your helping qualities*–without burning out. This is the challenge of caring.

The characteristics of empathy, helping motivations, commitment, and idealism make you particularly suited to helping others; but they may also be the very qualities that make it difficult for you to maintain appropriate boundaries. You must find a way to get close enough to identify the needs of the person you are helping, and yet remain far enough away that *their* problems don't become *yours*.

This is called "maintaining boundaries"–keeping an appropriate distance between you and the person you are helping.

If you are not close enough to the situation, you cannot accurately assess the person's needs and therefore correctly identify how you can best help. On the other hand, if you become too close, you may get so enmeshed that you lose your objectivity and may no longer be accurate in your assessments. How do we find this delicate balance and keep an appropriate distance?

Patients and families come to hospice with many needs. They enter into the relationship with the hospice staff at a time when they are emotionally vulnerable. Their focus is extremely limited as they attempt to come to terms with their new reality. Most likely, they have little knowledge of what to expect or how to handle practical concerns.

All of these things create an atmosphere of fear and anxiety that make them want to latch onto the hospice professionals as if they were their rescuers. We are, after all, the experts in this area. At least a part of them wants us to tell them exactly what to do so that everything will be okay. If only it were that simple. While it is true that we do have much experience and expertise to offer, we do not pretend to have the answer to every problem.

Even if we presumed to know exactly what would be right for each family in a given situation, we should not voice those opinions.

Our job is not to make choices for others, but to present them with options and explain them fully. We then must respect, support, and honor any choices made. Because we *do* care and because the families' needs are so great and their expectations so high, it is easy to see how a helper can become too involved in the situation.

The family *wants* to be rescued and we *want* to save them. It is sometimes difficult for us to see that the best way to help, ultimately, is to allow each patient and family their own experience and to stay within our role of education and support.

If we do otherwise, we rob them of the potential personal growth that often occurs as people walk this sacred journey. With the painful "good-byes" and "I love yous," with the tears and the overwhelming sense of loss, also may follow peace and spiritual enrichment. The opportunity to right past wrongs, to say precious final words to a loved one, to ensure that those being left behind will be taken care of, these are fleeting moments that inevitably shape our character and define our future. Who are we to impose our beliefs or values on an experience so uniquely personal and very private?

And it is not only "personal" growth that may occur. I have seen many instances of relationships that developed into a richer and deeper bond than had ever before been reached. Richard and Wanda are such an example.

At the time that Richard was diagnosed with cancer, his children had long since left the nest. He and his wife had spent thirty-five years together. Wanda raised their children and Richard built his business. After their children had grown and gone, Wanda and Richard found themselves to be virtual strangers.

Their responsibilities over the years, both domestic and business, had kept them too busy to maintain their relationship with each other. They had remained together physically but had grown emotionally distant. As Wanda shared with me, they had even discussed divorce a few times, but the long habit of living together was not altogether unpleasant.

As they pursued their separate interests, they became two people who shared only the same address. They drifted through life this way for many years, both on their own path, neither supporting nor tearing down the other.

When Richard's illness struck, he fought it with fervor for several years. He sought the advice of several of the country's finest oncologists. They offered him treatments, which he undertook until his body could no longer withstand the terrible side effects. Richard came home to die.

The surgeon who had originally diagnosed his cancer offered him the option of hospice care, with her as the attending physician. Richard and Wanda agreed, and hospice became involved.

Complicating matters for this couple was Wanda's state of health. She had many medical problems and was unable to care for Richard. Twenty-four-hour caregivers were hired, relieving Wanda of the physical strain and allowing her the energy to nurture Richard over the coming six months. Although blessed with many friends and neighbors, they restricted visitors to immediate family, their pastor, and the hospice staff.

Richard's illness placed new burdens on their relationship, but it also offered new opportunities. Richard was forced to accept assistance, rather than being the "strong" member of the family. Wanda was now in the position of taking primary responsibility for all decisions.

They had more time alone together than at any other time during their marriage. Slowly, hesitantly, they began to talk. They discovered, to their delight, that the love that had initially brought them together was still present, lying dormant under years of neglect. As they faced and tried to come to terms with their awful reality, that love grew.

At the time of Richard's death, Wanda spoke of the past six months as the most precious time of her life. It had in many ways been the most difficult, as well, but as she put it,

"I wouldn't have traded them for anything, bad as it was at times. If Richard had died suddenly in an accident, we would never have recaptured our love. Why did we wait so long? We wasted so much time!"

Part of what the hospice team was able to achieve with this family was to allow them to find their own way. The social worker and chaplain were available for support and did make occasional visits, but the blooming of this relationship was initiated and nurtured with no active intervention from the hospice team.

The team was able to convey their encouragement and support without interfering or intruding. Sometimes *staying out* of a situation is more difficult than *plunging in*, especially for those who have strong helping tendencies. Because most of our patients and families need so much from us, it is hard to sit back and let them handle the situation.

By not succumbing to the "knight in shining armor syndrome," we allow the patient and family to retain control over their situation. We also help ourselves by maintaining that appropriate distance. *Ideally, a helper is in a state of balance, able to become more emotionally involved when the situation calls for it and ready to pull back if that is what is necessary.*

When you become overly involved in a patient's situation, you may feel a great deal of personal distress. This is when you may blur the boundary lines. This can easily affect your ability to effectively work with a particular patient or family.

You may experience intense emotions–both positive and negative. You may feel exhilarated at the impact you are having on a person's life or that of his family. This intensity of feelings is exciting, but also exhausting. You may feel that you are the only person who can be effective with this patient and family.

When your coping resources become strained, you may try to reduce your involvement, either by setting healthy limits or by withdrawing emotionally and/or physically. Withdrawal, in this instance, can compound feelings of loss for a person who is already losing so much.

In an effort to help, we can lose sight of our own needs. It becomes critical to monitor ourselves and be alert for any sense that we may have gone too far. We must remember that we cannot be the *primary* source of psychosocial care for every patient we work with. We must remain outside the immediate situation, offering guidance and support, but not playing an active part.

This may mean giving up some of the gratification that comes from being in the spotlight with our shining armor. There is really no other way if we want to remain in this field. If we don't set limits, we will soon find that overload will eventually make us less available emotionally to the people we care for, at work *and* in our personal lives.

So what's the secret? Part of the answer lies in remembering that maintaining boundaries is a process, slightly different with each person we may work with. Depending upon a given situation and personality, we may feel more, or less, compelled to become involved.

For example, I would tend to be more highly involved with a patient who reminded me of my own beloved, deceased father-in-law than with a patient who had characteristics like the worst supervisor I have worked with. Just as each situation is different, so are the strategies each person may use to help himself or herself maintain an appropriate balance.

The following are suggested strategies you may want to adopt or adapt to your own comfort level.

Create a barrier between your personal and professional (helping) life

To provide balance in your life, you must learn to separate the workplace from the homeplace. The barrier you create could be a small symbolic act, such as simply turning off your pager or deliberately setting your work paraphernalia in the back seat of your car to await the next workday.

It could be a favorite song or phrase that reminds you to change gears. The technique you use does not matter. The important thing is to prevent problems on one side of your life from interfering with success and satisfaction in the other.

Develop a "stress-resistant" outlook

Seek to develop and nurture a sense of optimism and commitment. Be involved in life's activities that have meaning and interest for you. Look for challenges, not problems. Strive for a sense of control. This has a tendency to make us feel competent to cope with the challenge at hand.

Develop a support system

We all need to feel supported and appreciated for our efforts at work and at home. Because you are striving to keep these two worlds apart, you need different sources of support in both arenas. Only your family can provide the emotional nurturing that you need to feel loved and wanted at home.

Likewise, only your coworkers and peers can provide the kind of empathy, feedback, and encouragement that is essential to you as a "helper." And debriefing with your peers in a support group or more informal one-on-one interaction can give you an important sense that someone truly understands your feelings.

Maintain and enhance a sense of self-esteem

One way of feeling less threatened by a situation is to perceive yourself as being competent to deal with it. People who have high self-esteem tend to have less fear and cope better than those with low self-esteem. Build your confidence by always seeking to improve your skills. Keep up with the current literature, seek feedback on your performance, and so forth. Be accepting and forgiving of your errors but always strive to learn from them.

Reducing stress and maintaining balance in our lives requires that we take actions to change our internal and external worlds. It also requires that we open our hearts to ourselves. We must turn inward some of the same openness and compassion we show to others.

Boundaries for Primary Caregivers

A primary caregiver may be defined as anyone who assumes the responsibility for ensuring that the dying person's needs are fulfilled. This person may provide the care directly or may make arrangements for and supervise the care given by others. Although the physical burden may differ, the emotional burden is the same. Primary caregivers usually feel a strong sense of responsibility and may experience tremendous guilt, especially if circumstances prevent them from providing their loved ones' physical care.

Primary caregivers are experiencing a vast array of emotions, facing a situation that they most likely have not been taught to deal with. Their entire world seems as if it is spinning out of control. Caregivers may have had to put their jobs, their families, their entire lives on hold in order to fulfill their duties toward the dying persons. A natural response to feeling out of control is the tendency to attempt to "do it all," trying to be all things to all the people in their lives.

Until you have actually done the work, it is impossible to understand how difficult and laborious caregiving is. This is particularly true if one person is essentially responsible for twenty-four-hour care, including personal needs. Bathing, feeding, changing linens, all these activities require tremendous energy and stamina. Doing this on a twenty-four-hour basis is exhausting, even for someone who is *not* personally involved in the situation. The combination of physical fatigue and emotional turmoil can become overwhelming in a very short time.

Maintaining boundaries in this situation means knowing when you are approaching your limits of physical and emotional endurance. It also means being able to ask for assistance when you need it.

Caring for someone you love is one of the greatest gifts you can give that person. It is a tangible way of showing love, respect, and reverence. It is a personal challenge that many people feel strongly that they must do themselves, or it may not be done correctly. This intense sense of responsibility makes it difficult to accept help from others. Even if you believe they are competent to perform these tasks, you don't *want* them to.

As fatigue deepens and emotional responses are heightened, it may become difficult to know when you have reached your limits. It is imperative that you remain as vigilant about self-care as you are about caring for your loved one. In order to continue to help through the entire dying process, you must preserve physical and emotional resources. Whenever you feel overwhelmed, so tired you can't continue, angry, or frustrated, it is time to seek help.

Help is available from the hospice staff. They can arrange for *respite care*, relief from physical tasks so that the caregiver may rest. Respite care should be an available option. This can take several different forms, depending upon the needs of the patient and family.

If life expectancy is several weeks or months, respite on a regular basis should be arranged. A hospice worker, volunteer, friend, or other family member may stay with the dying person. The opportunity to spend a few hours running errands, getting your hair done, or taking a long walk may seem like a luxury you simply don't have time for or necessarily want. By caring for yourself, however, you are ultimately best helping your loved one. Most hospices have at least a volunteer who can stay with the patient, and some may provide skilled (nursing) care.

In some situations, leaving the person with others may not be acceptable or practical. The primary caregiver may not be comfortable with the idea of not being there every possible moment. Or the patient may insist that he not be left with anyone other than family.

If this is the case, at least consider allowing others to assist with everyday tasks such as grocery shopping or house cleaning. Many times you will hear friends and neighbors say, "If there's anything I can do to help, let me know…" This offer is usually sincere and prompted by their own helping tendencies. People want very much to help but are unsure how to do so without intruding.

Keep a perpetual list of tasks others can do, so that when this offer is made, you are ready to say, "Well, if you are going to the grocery store sometime soon, I could use a few items." The double benefit is that *you* are not so overwhelmed, and the person who performs this assignment feels good knowing that he or she has done something specific to assist you.

If the dying person has limited caregivers to share the responsibilities, those few may reach a point of absolute exhaustion. In this case, more than a few hours are needed for the family to rest. If hospice services are paid by Medicare, *inpatient respite care* in a nursing home or hospital should be offered by the hospice and can last as long as five days.

The decision to use inpatient respite care is one that should be reached together by the entire team of patient, family, attending physician, and hospice workers. The concept behind respite care is one that is fundamental to hospice philosophy: care of the *family* is equally as important as care of the patient.

The hospice team understands you have undertaken one of the most difficult roles of your life, that of caregiver to someone who is terminally ill. They admire and respect your desire to help your loved one die as peacefully as possible. With all of their knowledge and experience, they could never replace you. Like your friends and family, they are there to assist and support you. *Let them.*

---

[1]Kahil Gibran, *The Prophet* (New York: Alfred A. Knopf, 1971), p. 21.

CHAPTER SIX

The Dis-ease of Stress

Bobbie Crabb Jennings with John Spivey

*Learn to get in touch with the silence
within yourself,
And know that everything in this life has
a purpose.*

Elisabeth Kübler-Ross[1]

Three things are true of all end-stage illnesses. One, those involved–patient, caregivers, family members, and friends–will all experience stress at some point, and at some level. Two, our bodies respond to stress in predictable ways, whatever the cause may be. And three, there are simple things we can do to minimize the unhealthy effects stress has on our bodies, our minds, and our spirits.

Sadly, these "simple things" are rarely taught by healthcare providers and are, therefore, seldom recognized. We know by now that the death and dying experience is a process. And in the previous chapters, we have detailed how the process can control us because of a lack of education.

This chapter is designed to make you aware of just how much stress can impact your health, your attitude, and your behavior. When someone we love is dying, respite from stress is rare. While there may be no cure from stress during this time, we can learn to lessen its effects.

First, let's identify the term *stressors.* Stressors are primarily emotions, most of which are obvious, some of which are suppressed. Anxiety and fear, excitement and surprise, joy and sadness, anger and acceptance are all emotions that cause stress. We experience these daily, simply because we are alive.

These are common emotions, and we are accustomed to them. But they can still produce high levels of stress. They also trigger predictable, physical responses within our bodies. Although pain and fatigue are not considered emotions, they can elicit these same responses. Some of these responses are internal, such as increased blood pressure, increased heart rate, and increased respiration, all of which can suppress our immune system. This will eventually lead to more serious, life-threatening illnesses and for the terminally ill will also increase the severity of their condition.

Other responses are external and easily perceived *when and if* we are looking for them. As an example, go stand in front of a mirror, right now, and look at yourself. Observe your posture.

Are your shoulders uneven, tense? Or are they relaxed and level? Is your head forward or back? Is your chin tucked or protruding? Are you standing tall or are you slouched? Are you smiling or frowning? Is your forehead wrinkled, your eyebrows pinched? Are your hands clenched or relaxed? Are you breathing slowly and deeply, or shallowly and rapidly? Do your eyes sparkle or are they dull?

What would these various physical responses say about your mood, your stress and anxiety level, your pain? This is what we call "body language."

Now think of either the best or worst experience of your life. Replay that experience over in your mind, really *feel* that moment. Now look in the mirror. What does your body language reveal? Can you see how it might change when you move from anger to joy, from fear to sadness, or when you feel vital and alive as opposed to when you feel fatigued?

How often do we say we feel fine, that everything is okay, when just the opposite is true? It is at these times that our bodies and our words are not speaking the same language. When dealing with the terminally ill and their families, we know that they are experiencing many emotions, often all at once. If we are observant, body language can alert us to the fact that someone we care for is not okay. This is invaluable in determining how to interact with them.

Our pain, sadness, or anger will not magically disappear. Managing stress means listening to our body and "tuning in" to situations that create stress. It involves education, learning relaxation techniques like meditation and exercises that relieve tension.

The following is one such technique. From Dr. Herbert Benson, it is called "The Relaxation Response."

1. Sit quietly in a comfortable position.
2. Close your eyes.
3. Deeply relax all your muscles, beginning with your feet and progressing up to your face. Keep them relaxed.
4. Breathe through your nose. Become aware of your breathing. As you breathe out, say the word "One" silently to yourself. For example, breathe in, then out– "One." In and out–"One," and so on. Breathe easily and naturally.
5. Continue for ten to twenty minutes. You may open your eyes to check the time, but do not use an alarm. When you finish, sit quietly for several minutes, at first with your eyes closed and later with your eyes open. Do not stand up for a few minutes.
6. Do not worry whether you are successful in achieving a *deep* level of relaxation. Maintain a passive

attitude; permit relaxation to occur at its own pace. When distracting thoughts occur, try to ignore them by not dwelling on them and return to repeating "One." With practice, the response should come with little effort. Practice the technique once or twice daily, but not within two hours after any meal, since the digestive processes seem to interfere with elicitation of the relaxation response.[2]

One of the most important methods for dealing effectively with our stressors is developing a positive attitude. Have you ever noticed how a positive attitude puts you in control of your life? For those who are terminally ill, regaining some measure of control over their life, and death, means that they are not so much at the mercy of drugs and caregivers.

Research shows that stress reduces our immune system's ability to resist disease. When our immune system is compromised, even minor ailments can lead to more serious illnesses. Dr. Bernie Siegel, an oncologist, reports that patients with high levels of stress are more likely to develop cancer. He also found that cancer patients who dealt with their stress in a positive way survived longer, and in some cases even beat their cancer.

If stress can impact our immune system and contribute to illness, what happens when pain enters into the mix? Often, stress and physical pain go hand in hand. But there is little doubt that at some point, they will become kindred stressors. The "pain cycle" is a series of physiological events that can be set into motion in a number of ways. Consider the following scenario.

Someone smashes your finger in a door. Your first response is to grab your finger. Your heart rate and blood pressure shoot up, and you gasp for air as your body tenses. At this point, you might feel inclined to lash out at the offender. These are primary responses to pain. Eventually, the pain subsides, and you know that your finger will heal.

But let's say that, on some deeper level of which you are unaware, you have not resolved your anger toward the offender. In that case, over time, your heart rate and blood pressure continue to increase. But this is not something you notice because these problems commonly have no symptoms. However, all of this eventually leads to physical pain. The aching muscle tensions in your back and neck force you to seek medical attention. When asked, you cannot recall any specific trauma to your neck. Certainly, a smashed finger that healed months ago could not be the cause! But the very real pain you are experiencing is caused by the *emotional stress* of an incident that occurred long ago.

Unresolved emotions constantly influence our health, and our behavior. Anger is but one stressor that can set into motion an entire series of physiological events known as the "pain cycle."

The pain cycle can begin without an external cause. For example, Dorothy, a good friend of mine, had lived most of her life contented and happy. She was an emotionally well-balanced woman. Her son, however, was mentally impaired, and for several years before his death at the age of nineteen, she had served as his caregiver. She seemed to have accepted his loss and appeared to move on with her life.

Then she began to experience excruciating pain in her right leg. Her body language bespoke the unbearable pain she endured. Her posture was often rigid and fixed. She held her breath for periods of time. Her blood pressure and heart rate shot up; her respiratory rate nearly doubled.

Tension headaches were common, as were muscle spasms. She became anxious, fearful, angry, and sad. She was always exhausted. Before long, her "pain cycle" became a vicious cycle.

Doctors discovered a lesion at the root of a nerve in her right leg. Dorothy had cancer, and it had metastasized from her lungs to her lower spine. I wondered, was the cancer a response to the stress of caring for a disabled and dying son? We had no way of knowing for sure. Did the cancer cause the initial pain in her leg? Probably. Was the cancer responsible for increased blood pressure and heart rate, her rigid muscles and fixed posture? Yes, but indirectly. No doubt the pressure of the lesion on the nerve in her leg caused the pain that led to those responses.

Many of the emotions that can trigger stress were there—fear and anxiety, anger and sadness. In the end, Dorothy lost her ability to fight. I know that I lost my dear friend to the cancer and not to stress. But I wonder how much easier it might have been for her had she understood the critical role that stress plays in our lives and had the opportunity to deal with it effectively.

Are we at risk each and every time we become anxious or excited, sad or angry? No! Our body is designed to maintain itself and its systems in a state of balance or equilibrium. We are well equipped to handle the day in and day out stresses of living. Even an occasional traumatic event is easily confronted as long as we exercise and keep ourselves nourished and rested. Usually, we get into trouble only when *unresolved* emotions linger.

A much greater quality of life is attainable at all levels of our journey if we can just learn to maintain a more harmonious inner balance. To better understand how stress and the "pain cycle" can affect us, it might be helpful to briefly explore the major systems of the body and how they work together.

Our bones make up the *skeletal system* and give our body its shape. They also protect our vital organs, the heart, lungs, brain, and kidneys. Holding the bones together is the *muscular system* and its tendons and ligaments. Together, these two systems determine our shape and posture, and they allow us to move around.

Our *nervous system* is composed of the central nervous system—our brain and spinal cord and the peripheral nervous system—thirty-three pairs of nerves from the spinal cord filtering out to the trunk, arms, and legs. Functioning like an electrical system, the brain is the main breaker box and the "paired" nerves are the wires that send and receive messages to and from all living tissue. The nerves provide a connection from the brain to every part of the body.

The brain receives information from our senses: sight, sound, odor, feel, by way of the sensory nerves. Every time a sensory nerve is irritated or injured, it sends a signal to the brain. Once the sensation is received in the brain, it responds by sending a message to the muscles and tissues via the motor nerves and allows us to take action.

Also working together are the heart and lungs, which comprise the *cardiopulmonary system.* The heart is a muscle that pumps blood from the lungs to all parts of the body via the arteries, carrying nutrition and oxygen to every living cell. Waste products, such as carbon dioxide, are returned to the lungs through the veins. During normal breathing, oxygen is taken into the lungs and is exchanged for carbon dioxide.

Arteries, veins, and nerves are bundled neatly together in a sheath. They run through muscles and across joints and have small branches that go to all *living tissue* throughout the body. Since blood vessels and nerves run through the muscles, whenever we tense up, whether from stress or pain, the muscles squeeze the vessels and nerves.

If nerves get pinched hard enough, a sensation of pain is sent to the brain, and the body automatically tenses. When muscles put force on the arteries and veins, the heart has to pump harder and faster to push the blood through these compressed vessels. This can cause heart rate and blood pressure to increase.

Over time, untreated muscle tension and pain can cause a build up of waste products in our muscles. This hinders blood flow and causes more pain. Thus, we tense, hold our breath, and compress our nerves and vessels; as this happens, blood pressure, heart rate, and respiration rate rise.

The "pain cycle" begins.

Let's talk about posture. When you are tired or in pain, it is normal to slump. When you do, the lungs are unable to fully expand and take in oxygen. You must increase your rate of breathing to get enough oxygen in the blood to supply all your living tissue. This requires your heart to pump a larger volume of blood, and as it does, heart rate and blood pressure rise as well.

The explanation just presented should elicit a mental picture of how all of this works. Stress precipitates stress, which only causes more stress. Now that you are better prepared to identify the signs of stress and its effects, how can you minimize or break down the pain cycle?

Breaking Down the Pain Cycle

The following exercises are designed for anyone, but especially for a caregiver or patient. Remember, by observing facial expressions and recognizing tone of voice, muscle tension, breathing patterns, and posture, you can identify stress. Upon doing so, there are many things you can do to make a difference. And regardless of your physical condition, many of these techniques can help you to minimize the effects of stress.

RELAXATION. Breathing and posture go hand in hand. This means finding a position that is comfortable, one that allows all of the body systems to work at peak efficiency, whether sitting, standing, or reclining. This position, or posture, is called "optimal alignment." Avoid positions that compromise body functions, such as slumping, crossed arms or legs, and frequent bending at the joints.

From the "mirror" exercise, you understand how easily your alignment can become distorted when you are in pain or are stressed. You have also seen how tension can be relieved when using relaxation exercises such as Benson's breathing techniques.

Now let's try it. Lift your chest, tuck in your chin, and breathe in slowly through your nose. *Feel* your chest expand. *Feel* your body begin to relax.

Remember, as you lift your chest and allow more air into your lungs per breath, your heart won't have to beat so fast to get that good oxygen to your body's cells. Be careful, though! You may get dizzy from so much oxygen. You will *feel* your tense muscles relax because muscle tension will not occur while you are breathing so deeply. Once you let go of tension, you will let go of pain, for you are no longer compressing the nerves that cause it.

The next time you observe a loved one in pain, ask if you can take hold of their hand and gently massage it, softly suggesting, "Let me help you relax. Breathe with me. Let's take some deep breaths, slowly, in through your nose. Now lift your chest. Slowly again, blow the air out through your mouth and then let your chest down. Good. Pause. Now do it again...slowly...always slowly...in...and out."

When a state of relaxation is achieved, you will notice it in their softened face and a lessening of their muscle tension.

Hopefully, you can see the importance of being in touch with your emotions and how your body responds to them.

An easy reminder is to STOP, LOOK, and LISTEN.

> STOP...Think about your day. Did you take time for you? Did you notice the green of the trees, the clouds borne on the winds, a smile on a child's face?
>
> LOOK...Have you looked at yourself lately? Really looked? Do you feel the way you look? Is this a good thing?
>
> LISTEN...Listen to your body, to your voice, to your breathing, to your heartbeat, to your emotions, to your *stressors.*

Attitude is everything. Whether you are a caregiver or one who is terminally ill, you have choices. In this chapter, we have discussed the causes of stress, how it affects your body, and how to reduce stress. We encourage each of you to take time during the day to examine how you are feeling and to become attuned to your body. Then try some of the exercises found in appendix A. They will help.

Ralph Waldo Emerson said that what lies behind us and what lies before us are tiny matters compared with what lies within us. In the end, being in touch with your emotions is simply being in touch with yourself.

---

[1]Julia Cameron, as quoted in *The Artist's Way* (New York: G.P. Putnam's Sons, 1992), p. 45.

[2]Herbert Benson and Eileen Stuart, *The Wellness Book: The Comprehensive Guide to Maintaining Health and Treating Stress Related Illness* (Boston: New England/Deaconness Hospital and Howard University Press, 1992), p. 45f.

CHAPTER SEVEN

If...

Denise Glavan

You who live in the shelter of the Most High,
who abide in the shadow of the Almighty,
will say to the LORD, "My refuge and my
fortress;
my God, in whom I trust."

Psalm 91:1–2

When Sarah was referred to me, she had recently been told that she had six months to live. Suddenly faced with death, she did not want to deal with it. At first, she acted as if nothing was wrong. She told her children, ages nine and fourteen, that she was fine.

As her condition worsened, however, it became plain that this was not true. Gradually, she lost the ability to speak and to eat by mouth. Finally, the only way she could communicate was through pen and paper. When she answered

66

the phone, her attempt at hello became a deep, guttural sound: "Huuuuh!"

When I called to set up an appointment, her nine-year-old son answered the phone.

"Huuuuh!" he said, imitating his mother. This was an immediate red flag. He was struggling to make sense of an unbearable reality. He could not deal with his mother's condition in a healthy way because no one had been honest with him.

I spent many hours talking with the children. But, since Sarah would not allow a discussion of her impending death, there was just so much I could do. My hands were tied. She told me repeatedly that she did not want her children to know; she did not want them to worry. And the children went along with her charade. When asked, they always said, "Mother's just fine." Naturally, all this did was multiply their fears.

Time wore on and Sarah could no longer communicate even by writing. The children's confusion and anger began to find outlets. All were destructive. Her son internalized his feelings and never caused a problem. He always did as he was told. He became the perfect son. Inside, however, his emotions and fears consumed him.

Her daughter became openly angry and defiant. She had boys over at all times of the day and night. She began failing in school. Since they were not allowed to talk about their feelings, both were mortally afraid.

If, today, you found out you had only six months to live, what would you do? What if it was only three months? How about a week? Forty-eight hours? What would you do? Might you be like Sarah and deny that anything was wrong with you?

Would you gather all your loved ones together to say good-bye? Would you throw caution to the wind and suddenly try to do all the things you've always wanted to do? Would you make amends for the wrongs you have committed?

Would you spend your time trying to deal openly with the issues of death? Would you work to get your financial house in order? Prepare your will? Would you continue to do the same things you are doing now? Or would you do nothing at all?

What if it was your spouse, your child, or your parent?

A lot of questions, I know. But these are questions we seldom ask ourselves until actually confronted with death. I was given the opportunity to ask these questions to members of Peace Lutheran Church, where I was teaching the material found in this book.

All agreed that losing a child would be hardest, because our children are supposed to outlive us. Our natural instinct is, of course, to protect our children from harm, especially death.

But were it they who were dying, they said that their responses would vary. They also acknowledged that their responses toward each family member would be different.

Consider how Sarah dealt with her situation. By not allowing a discussion of her illness or impending death, she prevented her children from being given a means with which to cope. Denial is never a healthy solution, though this is where many begin. We can alleviate much, but not all, of our pain and suffering by educating ourselves. If we do not, the experience can simply be too hard on us.

We must remember that we have a right to our feelings, whatever they may be. They are not to be discounted, because when we discount our feelings, we are discounting ourselves. Feelings are neither good nor bad, they just are. They are a part of us. We may try to hide our feelings, but eventually they will find an outlet.

Often they are *acted out*. This is when you take your anger, hurt, fear, or frustration out on others, yourself, even, and sometimes especially, on the ones you love. This is exactly what Sarah's children did. Learning to acknowledge your feelings can be very hard. Experienced hospice counselors can help you work through your feelings. They can help you face your own death or come to terms with losing someone you love.

As we accept that nothing can be done to fix our situation, we will need support. This is what hospice is all about. Support can come from any member of the hospice team. The nurse, chaplain, social worker, home health aide, or volunteer is skilled in terminal care. Support can also come from friends and family. If you find yourself in such a role, you have the potential to stabilize a chaotic situation.

Remember, feelings are ever present when people are faced with death. Listening is key, as is your very presence. Be careful what you say. A word or phrase that might comfort you might have the opposite effect on one who is dying or a member of his family.

One day, I was with a family in the ER. I was there to offer support to a woman who had just lost her baby to Sudden Infant Death Syndrome. The child was six weeks old. The mother clutched her baby tightly and asked, "Why did God take my baby? I need my baby!"

Just at that moment, her grandmother walked into the room. She shook her head sadly and said, "Honey, God needs another rose in heaven." The mother screamed, "No! I need my baby more! God does not need another rose. He has enough! *I need my baby more!* " The poor grandmother thought her words would comfort. But they did not.

Once, while serving as a chaplain at Baptist Medical Center in Oklahoma City, I was present as a woman gave birth to her baby. It was stillborn.

"I guess God wanted another angel in heaven," she said softly. "At least I had my baby for nine months. I do not know why, but I just know that God will give me the strength to go on." Though her words were similar to the grandmother's, somehow these words comforted her.

Another hospice patient of mine was a 27-year-old man with AIDS. A minister said to his mother, "If you have enough faith, if you have faith as small as a mustard seed, miracles can occur."

When I introduced myself, his mother asked, "Why is God punishing me? My minister told me that if I had enough faith, a miracle would occur. I have been praying and praying, and still my son is not cured. Why? I have faith. I do!" She had reached a breaking point because she felt it was all her fault. It took many long hours to help this woman realize that God was not punishing her, that God loved her and her son.

Because of ignorance, it is our tendency to think in these ways, to respond to tragedy with such comments. These statements may be comforting to some, but to others they can be inappropriate and dangerous.

Certainly, we do not intend to hurt another with our words. Tread carefully. If you do not know what to say, *then say nothing.* Listen. Just listen. Your presence can itself be a comfort.

The following statements are often said with the best of intentions but have the potential to hurt:

God wants another angel in heaven.

God needs you more.

Everything will be okay.

You are going to have to get tough.

You have to face this, buck up and deal with it.

It is not our job, or anyone else's, to make a dying person and his or her family accept what is going on. Nor is it our responsibility to make it better. We cannot fix this. All we can do is be there, offer our support, and walk with them on this very painful journey.

Another patient of mine had just been released from the hospital to a nursing home. I walked into his room, a room filled with flowers and get well cards. Hanging on his bedroom wall was a huge banner with the words, "Get well! We love you."

"Hello," I said. "My name is Denise. I am the chaplain with hospice."

"Hello," his wife returned. "I'm glad to meet you. This is my husband, Tom. He is getting better all the time. I just know he is. He can't leave me. He takes care of me. He's everything to me. Everything will be fine. First, we got him out of the hospital, and soon, when he is stronger, I'm going to take him home."

Obviously, she was in a strong state of denial.

"I'm glad to meet you too," I replied. It was not my job to leap in and try to make her accept the hard fact that her husband was dying. So, I asked careful questions and listened.

"Tell me what is wrong with your husband."

"Why, nothing. As I said, he's getting better."

I listened as she continued to try to convince herself, and me, how much his condition was improving. And that's all I did. Because at that point, that was what she needed.

Often, a dying person and his or her family are at different levels of acceptance. And we may find ourselves trying to force one another to face death and accept it before we're ready. And there are those who cannot face death until it actually occurs. And this is okay. If we cannot force a person to deal with death before she is ready, what can we do?

The following statements further demonstrate compassionate and sensitive ways to communicate without forcing your agenda on those who are not ready.

DON'T SAY:	"You should accept that Sam is going to die."
SAY:	"It sounds like you are really hurting." (Or: angry, frustrated, depressed)
DON'T SAY:	"You should stop crying. You have to face this."
SAY:	"It's okay to cry."
DON'T SAY:	"You should be thankful that we have this time together. You're feeling sorry for yourself."
SAY:	"I'm here. We don't have to talk. I'll just sit here and be with you."
DON'T SAY:	"Accept it. She's going to die. Complaining does no good."

SAY: "Do you feel like talking? Do you want to tell me about it?"

DON'T SAY: "How are you feeling today?" (It's a given that they do not feel well. No one wants to die.)

SAY: "How are things today?"

Death causes our deepest emotions to emerge. Everyone will deal with it in his or her own way, and in his or her own time. There is no need to force people to deal with death before they are ready.

IF... today, you found out you had only six months to live, or were it someone you loved, what would you do?

What would you say?

How would you act?

CHAPTER EIGHT

Grief and Bereavement

John Spivey
with
Shelly Hartwick

What will I do now that you are gone?

We grieve. We grieve because we have lost, or are losing, something very dear and precious, and in the midst of our grief, it is hard to see our way out. *Sure,* we tell ourselves, *things will get better,* but then memories intrude and our hearts begin to break all over again. It *feels* as if nothing will ever be the same again.

And even though we may feel as if we are dying inside, grieving means that we are very much alive. In fact, if we did not grieve, we would be dead inside.

Up to this point, we have described many instances of loss and the subsequent feelings of grief. For many, grief is just a word. Someone we love has died and we are sad, mournful. We shed tears and then we move on. After all, this is America, the land of the busy, the land of denial, and we simply don't have the time (or could it be that we don't know how) to grieve.

Whether you have time or not, whether you want to or not, *you will grieve.* If you try to avoid the process, nevertheless, your grief will seek, and find, a less healthy outlet. As you will see, when you allow yourself to grieve, you will find the path to healing and recovery.

Elisabeth Kübler Ross describes five basic stages of grief. They are:

DENIAL   We are in shock. We are numb. We refuse to comprehend that this is happening.

ANGER   When denial can no longer be maintained, we become angry. *Why?* We rage. It is an appropriate question. We even rage at the people who are dying.

BARGAINING   "If only...," we begin. "If only, dear God, you will allow me to live long enough to see my first grandchild..." or "If only you will let my loved one live a little longer, I won't ask for anything more." God has been known to participate in the bargaining process. God listens. And, of course, it never hurts to ask.

DEPRESSION   To say that depression is normal is a bit of an understatement. It's hard to get out of bed, hard to find the energy to want to go on. You are losing someone you love. But your loved one is losing everything.

ACCEPTANCE   You know that you will survive. You still hurt, to be sure, and your grief will not be any less intense when death does arrive. But it is expected.

The odd thing about grief is that you may or may not experience these feelings in the order as listed above. Just when you feel as if you have conquered depression, denial might sneak right back in. Or you may feel anger and depression while in denial. Since grief is a continuous process, you must work your way through these stages *at your own pace, and in your own time.* Most importantly, remember that each stage is necessary, natural, and an integral part of the healing process.

There is another feeling we often encounter when someone we love is dying, and that is one of helplessness. The following letter expresses the various thoughts of many in this position:

I know this is awkward for you. You are frightened, confused, and you may not know what to say. Let me help you just as I know you want to help me. As my death nears, there are things I need. But mostly, *I need you.* Please don't avoid me. There is a kind of "loneliness" that descends upon only those who are dying. Do not be afraid to visit because, often, this "loneliness" is more than I can bear. And when you visit, do not be in a hurry. Be patient, loving, and nonjudgmental.

I need someone with the courage to let me talk, and I need someone with the courage to *listen.* Allow me to lead the conversation in the direction I want to go and please—just *listen.* I might want to talk about my life. If I do, help me by *listening* to my endless, repetitive stories. I might need to talk about my illness or my death. Don't let this bother you. *I'm just trying to make sense of it all.*

I would like you to think about this...*listening is a privilege.* It might be easier for you if you take a moment to put yourself in my shoes. When I ask you to listen, and you start giving me advice, you have not done what I asked. When I ask you to listen, and you begin to tell me why I shouldn't feel this way, you are trampling on my feelings. When I ask you to listen, and you feel you have to do something to solve my problem, you have failed me, strange though that may seem.

All I ask is that you *listen.* Hear me. Advice is cheap. A quarter will get you Dear Abby and Billy Graham in the same newspaper. To some extent, I can do for myself; I am not helpless. I may be discouraged, I may be faltering, but I am not helpless. *I know you mean well, but when you do something for me that I can do for myself, you contribute to my fear and weakness.*

When you accept that I feel what I feel, no matter how irrational, then I can stop trying to convince you, and we can get down to the business of understanding what's behind this irrational feeling. When that's clear, the answers are obvious and I won't need advice. Perhaps that's how prayer works. God doesn't give advice or try to fix things. In this respect, God is mute. *God just listens. And God lets us work things out for ourselves.* Won't you please do the same for me?

Maybe I don't need to talk at all. If you ask, I will tell you. Perhaps we could sit and simply enjoy the silence together. Sometimes silence creates emptiness. Sometimes silence creates opportunities. *Listen to the sound that isn't.*

Bring me a warm smile, a positive attitude. I can handle it and besides, it's catching. Talk to me of the future, of tomorrow, of next week, or next year. It's okay. *Hope is so important to me.*

Help me feel good about my looks. *Touch me.* A simple squeeze of my hand is like a great big hug. Allow me to be cheerful if that is how I feel or to weep if that is how I feel. On the other hand, it's okay if you cry too. It tells me that you care.

There's something you should know: I hear better than you think I do. Don't whisper out in the hall or in another room. The hospice nurse will tell you that even if I am in a coma, I may be able to hear you. If I am tired, tell me to close my eyes and rest. But don't leave. Time is a luxury we no longer enjoy. *Stay with me and hold my hand.*

Remember how it feels when everyone is quietly working at opposite ends of the house? You know they are there, and this is a comfort. Now think of how it feels when you know the house is empty. *Many times, the most powerful and comforting gift you can give is you.* It is called "the ministry of presence."

I need you to give me the help I ask for, not the help you think I should have. Tell me what you can do for me and then, if I agree, do it. I need you to tell me when you do *not* want to do something. Don't allow me to become a tyrant in my last days. *I need you to be honest, for this helps me to be honest.*

Frequently, I will want to talk about God. Let's share our faiths. Pray with me, and pray for me. Sometimes I might ask, Why is this happening to me? Those who are dying often feel as if they are being punished, so be gentle. *Don't tell me what you believe, ask what I believe.* And don't worry if I become angry with God. In fact, I may need you to help me understand that it is all right to express such anger.

Return when you say you will. If you cannot, call and tell me when you are coming. *Always say goodbye.* It gives me the option to tell you that I might not see you again. And do not forget to tell me that you love me if you do.

Spend time with those who are caring for me. They are probably tired. They may be dealing with feelings of guilt, too, because they cannot make my illness go away. Or they may be angry at others who could not make it go away. They may even be angry with me because I am ready to die, and they do not want me to.

Finally, my friend, remember, you do not have to solve my problems or give me answers. *All you really need to do is be here.*

Such explanations are necessary only when we fail to comprehend the profound significance death has on our lives.

Were we to heed the voice of one who is dying, might we not ease their passage? Were we to do so, might we not ultimately lessen our pain and our grief?

When we are faced with losing someone we love, what is the most grievous thing that can happen? Death itself? Not necessarily. If this book teaches anything, it is the hope that death should not be perceived in such a way. Perhaps the most grievous thing is that we do not feel free to express ourselves in this most emotional of times.

There is an old saying: it is not the destination that counts, but the journey. Seldom has this had more meaning than here, on this sacred journey. You might wonder, how do we *not* focus our attention constantly and intently on the destination? Sometimes there is something to be said for living in the moment. And it is moments like these that can show us, more clearly than anything else, that life has meaning.

———

At some point, if we are fortunate, we will have the opportunity to say goodbye to our loved one. Have you ever considered what you might say? If you have never been there, you have no way of appreciating just how short that time might be, or just how much you will want to say, or how you will feel. This moment, *right now,* might be a good time to think about such an occasion.

No man or woman can accurately articulate the joy of childbirth. You have to experience it as a parent. This is a *life* experience. Occasions such as these are rare in our lifetime; they are, in fact, "holy." And nothing can completely prepare you for it. Such is the experience of a final farewell.

What words would honor your loved one? What words would express your regrets? What words would complete unfinished business? And what words would put you both at peace?

Don't neglect to say good-bye.

———

And so, someone we love has died. Why does emptiness feel so heavy? Why does aimlessness seem our only direction?

We may reside for a while in disbelief. We may be unable to concentrate. Our chest or throat may feel tight. We are overly considerate to those who seem uncomfortable or do not know what to say to us. Or maybe we are not considerate. We have the need to remember and to talk of our memories. And all the while, we sense that our loved one is near.

It all feels so unnatural, and yet, just the opposite is true. We are not going crazy. We are responding normally and naturally to the loss of our loved one. While grief is as unique and individual as we ourselves are, these are *common* feelings. For this reason, we can share our grief with each other and help each other for a while. In the end, however, we must find our own way. How do we do this? How. . .

In their book, *How to Survive the Loss of a Love,* Melba Colgrove and Harold Bloomfield tell us:

> Although you may be frightened by it, be with your pain. Feel it. Lean into it. You will not find it bottomless. It is an important part of the healing process that you be with the pain, experience the desolation, feel the hurt. Don't deny it or cover it or run away from it. Be with it. Hurt for awhile. See pain as not hurting, but as healing.[1]

As Cindy suggested in her chapter on boundaries, listen to your heart. It's okay to cry; we *should* cry. It's okay to be angry; perhaps we *should* be angry. It's okay to do nothing; we *should* do nothing, for a while.

Ultimately, grief requires us to be participants in its process. This can be a very scary proposition because it means risking that very same heart that contains a lifetime of deep feelings that many of us seem happy to avoid. Maybe we sense that, when someone we love dies, grief is forever. And, on some level, perhaps it is.

The *process* of grief first requires us to acknowledge our loss, and then to acknowledge the pain of our loss. From here, we can begin to remember, even reexperience, our relationship with our loved one. Now, we can let go of our old attachments to them because we recognize and accept that they are gone. We adapt, and as we move on, we establish a new relationship, even though they are no longer with us.

Throughout this process, you will be developing a new sense of yourself, reflecting the many changes that have happened to you with your loss.

We must understand, however, that the *process* occurs differently for each individual; and for each individual, this will happen in his or her own time.

Don't rule out the value of a support group. Groups are safe places to discuss your feelings with others who have been there or who are there now. Postpone major, life-altering decisions for at least one year; this is a unique time in your life, a time for healing. Write down your deepest feelings in a journal—*now*; it will be a treasure to you later.

Above all, remember: you are not alone. Others you know have been there. They will be there to help you share the load if you let them. Do not deny them the opportunity.

The bereaved will need time alone, time when nothing, absolutely nothing, is expected of them. While they will share their grief among themselves, another natural resource for this is their friends. A family will need friends to ask about them and help them cope; friends who will listen to them without judgment; friends who will not try to rescue them; friends to help them make present and future plans.

As a friend, consider the following:

You cannot take away their pain. Do not try to explain away their loss in religious or philosophical terms, such as "Your mother is in a far better place now" or "This is God's will." At this time, the only place they want their loved one is with them, here and now. With that in mind, do not let your own sense of helplessness keep you from reaching out. Call and visit frequently, if they allow it.

Simply let your genuine concern and caring show. The bereaved *need* to talk about their loss. Encourage expressions of grief. But when you do, expect to encounter volatile reactions. *Grief knows no right or wrong way to express itself.* Grief is selfish. It is all-encompassing, affecting thoughts, emotions, actions, and physical well-being. It leaves little energy to attend to self or others.

The great need of those who are mourning is to have their feelings of fear, anger, sadness, guilt, despair, or even apathy accepted *without judgment.* They have earned the right to grieve, and no one has the right to take their pain away.

Children and Grief

If adults struggle with the process of grief, what goes on in the mind of a child? There is no age limit to grief.

Perhaps the most effective and realistic place to begin to change how our culture deals with death is at home, with our children. The experience of death is one that most of us probably try to shield our children from. If, from the beginning, we taught them the truths espoused in this book, we might ward off the fear that follows us in adulthood.

Not so long ago, the family unit commonly consisted of several generations of one family—all living under the same roof. Not only were children more aware of aging, illness, and death; they were encouraged to be a part of the rituals surrounding these. Families did not fear death. It was considered to be a natural part of life.

Children are rarely exposed to death now because people do not die at home anymore. We die in hospitals or nursing homes. Also, since we are a society constantly on the move, families are scattered geographically. Often, it is not logistically or economically possible to attend a funeral.

Today, instead of including our children in the death and dying experience, many of us try to protect them from it. In the attempt to shield them, however, we are not protecting them at all. We simply add to the fear and confusion children surely feel when they lose someone they love.

We must not make the mistake of thinking that they do not feel the same emotions adults do, albeit on a different level. We cannot protect them from loss, nor should we. Just as we cannot completely protect them from life itself, we cannot protect them from death. Wise guardians include their children in the experience of death, thus preparing them for life.

For just a moment, put yourself in a child's shoes. Your grandfather has died. You have been told that he has gone away to a better place, or maybe that he is now with God. But you didn't get to see him leave or say good-bye. Being a child, you think, "Papa always kisses me good-bye. He will come back, maybe tomorrow. And when he does, we will go fishing again!"

A day or so passes, but Papa doesn't come back. No one talks to you and everyone is sad. You may be a little frightened now. Somehow, you know to stay out of the way and be quiet. Everyone goes to the funeral (whatever that is), but they do not take you. You are left alone, with many confusing thoughts and unanswered questions.

We should simply be honest with our children when talking about death, but we need to talk to them on their level. We should do this according to their *developmental* age, not their *chronological* age.

Six years of age and under

With children below the age of six, adults must be absolutely clear on what they are *saying* and on what is being *heard*. This group understands you in the "literal" sense. So when we tell a five-year-old that Papa went on a trip, she believes that Papa went on a trip—and he is coming back.

There is the story of the little girl taken to a counselor after the death of her mother. She is obviously angry.

The counselor asks her, "Are you angry with your father?"

"No," the little girl replies.

"Are you angry with your mother?"

"No."

"Can you tell me who you are angry with?"

"I'm angry with the *angels*!" she snaps.

"My goodness, child, why?" the counselor asks.

"Because Daddy said that the angels came and took Mommy to heaven, and now they won't bring her back!"

A child at this age takes your words at face value. Simple and protective explanations such as "She's gone bye-bye" can create confusion and anxiety. The result could be that they might not want to let you out of their sight, fearing that you might go "bye-bye" and not return.

A child below the age of six rarely comprehends the *finality* of death. After all, Bugs Bunny never really dies. It is not until the age of eight that the concept of finality is literally understood. But even though this group cannot quite grasp the concept, when we tell them that someone they love has died, they accept that something has happened. Their pain will be in the *separation.*

Six years of age and beyond

A child over the age of six is developmentally tackling the concept of life and death, living and nonliving things. They develop what seems to be a morbid curiosity of death. For instance, one might stick a pin in the back of an insect and then watch how far it crawls until it is dead. In their own way, they are trying to grasp the reality of death.

Adults may find this behavior strange and react with revulsion. As a result, they might send the message that death is a terrible thing and not to be talked about. In fact, this is a perfect time to begin discussing the concept. And as we answer their many questions, we must not forget to *listen* to what they have to say.

Around eight years of age, the concept of finality really begins to sink in. For that reason, it is not uncommon for a child who has lost a loved one before this age to reexperience the loss at this time.

Children's grief has many dimensions. They may include the following:

AN APPARENT LACK OF FEELINGS. Moments after learning of the death, you might find them out in the backyard playing merrily, as if nothing at all has happened. This may be confusing to adults, but the children may be experiencing emotional shock. This is a protective mechanism; it is nature's way of helping them cope. By detaching themselves from the pain, children temporarily escape from the reality of losing a loved one. Be supportive and accepting of this behavior.

REGRESSION. You may have noticed that during stressful times, children's behavior will regress. They may wish to be held and rocked; they may ask a parent to tie their shoes; they may fear separation from mom and dad. This behavior may shock parents because it hasn't been exhibited in years. Don't let this bother you; regression in bereaved children is almost always temporary.

BIG MAN SYNDROME. "You take good care of your Mommy. You're the man of the house now." This, of course, would represent the opposite of regression. Well-intentioned though this may be, it sends the wrong message to a child. In order to replace the person who is gone, children may begin to express adult behavior before their time. No child should have to grow up this quickly.

Often, adults find themselves more comfortable dealing with children on this level, thus reinforcing this message. In the end, attempting to meet the inappropriate expectations of adults may damage a child's self-esteem and self-identity. Finally, children may unconsciously adopt this syndrome as a symbolic means of trying to keep their loved one alive. Remember, deal with children on *their* level.

ACTING OUT. Generally speaking, "acting out" is just another way in which children express themselves. In this case, they might be saying, "I'm hurting too." This may manifest itself as anger, resentment, and blame. But behind these often explosive emotions are the primary feelings of pain, helplessness, frustration, and fear.

Strong emotional outbursts are normal. Acting out is a reaction to feelings of insecurity, and it returns to them a sense of strength and control. Their pain and grief is often exhibited through acting out, and this can be difficult during a very trying time. Though we adults are dealing with our pain as well, we must be sensitive to them.

LOSS AND LONELINESS. Depression in children may manifest itself as a general lack of interest in themselves, a change in appetite or sleeping patterns, nervousness, an inability to enjoy life, and low self-esteem. School grades may also drop, since the ability to concentrate is also affected.

RECONCILIATION. This is the recognition that life will be different without their loved one. There is no timetable for the process of grief. Reconciliation will depend on such factors as the child's age, personality, social environment, and relationship to the person who has died.

Children return to stable eating and sleeping patterns. They feel a renewed sense of well-being and an increased ability to enjoy life again. And finally, they recognize the finality of death. But events like holidays and birthdays may invite grief to stop by; the various stages of grief may sneak back into their lives at these times. It is normal for adults, and it is equally normal for children.

Remember, a child in grief is still a child. Parents hope that their children will live a full and happy life. We want to protect them from the harsh realities of the world. And so we might say, "They will grow up soon enough. Let them be kids."

But the hard truth is that life is only complete with both happiness and pain. Such is our existence on Earth. If children are to grow into healthy adults, we must allow for this. We must give them permission to feel their pain and provide them ample room to express themselves.

They are stronger than we give them credit for. So are we.

---

[1]Melba Colgrove, Harold Bloomfield, and Peter McWilliams, *How To Survive the Loss of a Love* (Los Angeles, Calif.: Prelude Press, 1991), p. 30.

CHAPTER NINE

The Gift of You

Ann Wink with John Spivey

I am grateful for all the positive things that have been a result of Dad's illness and death: my children being able to be with Dad at the end of his life and for them to have closure; for my brother and me to have time together, alone, as brother and sister, and with my Mom and Dad, as a family; to be able to help Mom when she needed me; to have been able to care for Dad when he needed me most; and finally, to tell him how much I loved him.

I am also grateful that I had an opportunity to write all that I remembered of those seventeen days down on paper. At times, I had to stop writing because of the pain and then it was very difficult to get started again. But I believe that "living" the pain is the only way to get through it.

From the journal of Ann Wink, "Dad's Journey Toward Death."

My father died on March 30, 1994, after a long battle with cancer. I worked with a hospice at the time, and yet, my experience with death and dying did not make his passing any easier. During this time, there were those who volunteered to help, and I have never forgotten them.

Webster's defines *volunteer* as a person who enters into service of his own free will. Defined this way, it is easy to see why a volunteer would be such a blessed member of the hospice team. Volunteers will tell you that they feel privileged to work with the terminally ill and their families. And though Medicare *requires* hospices to use volunteers, they remain a select class of people freely offering their time and talents out of a sincere desire to help and learn.

The volunteer becomes a part of the team and actually works with the paid professional in establishing the plan of care. You may wonder what a volunteer could possibly do for a patient and family that a nurse, chaplain, or social worker could not do. In this chapter, I will share with you the volunteer's journey.

As a director of volunteers, my first task was to identify people's motivations and needs prior to placement. This was imperative if I was to put the right people with the right families. By not doing so, I risked losing precious time, time with a patient who may have very little of that left. And after the intensive training, a volunteer is too valuable a member of the team not to be appropriately placed.

Some volunteers choose to begin their work in an administrative position, helping secretaries and patient care managers in the office. But many, because they have personally suffered a loss, desire direct patient contact. Assuming the role of bereavement volunteer is a common and meaningful way for one to become involved.

Motivations generally fall into three areas: a curiosity about death and the process, a willingness to give back, based on their own experience with loss, or simply a desire to help.

The story of Toni is a unique and beautiful one. But then, all of my volunteers were unique and beautiful. Toni was dying when she volunteered. She was only twenty-two years old. Suffering from congestive obstructive pulmonary disease, she had been in and out of hospitals all her young life, and her physical appearance testified to this.

Her neck and face were scarred from numerous invasive procedures and she coughed constantly, as if from a persistent cold. For this reason, people tended to shy away from her at first, that is, until they got to know her. Even though she was dying, she would be an active patient care volunteer until only months before her death.

We worked together for two years, and seldom have I encountered one so willing to help. I understood her *motivation* for volunteering–she wanted to help. But Toni was a very private person, and it would be a long time before I fully understood her *need*. Shortly before she died, however, she shared this with me.

As we sat and talked one day, she said, "Ann, I believe I know what it will be like to die. I needed to understand this as best I could, because I was afraid." Then, with a tranquility that moved me deeply, she said, "I know now that it's okay."

Like so many of us, Toni feared the unknown that death represented to her. By investing a part of her life in helping others, when her time drew near, she found herself more at peace.

Lois was another unique volunteer with whom I was privileged to work. She was fighting breast cancer. Like Toni, she had not yet come to terms with her mortality but wished to help others who had. But instead of direct patient contact, she chose to contribute her talents in arts and crafts.

Lois was a real whiz at creating special gifts for our patients. As time passed, she became comfortable with the staff and their mission. While designing and constructing simple yet beautiful presents and remembrances, she gradually learned to accept her own prognosis. As we have discussed, this is no small task for anyone.

Still, I did not encourage her to venture out into patient care. I waited. Finally, she volunteered to see a patient. It was at this very time that Lois' condition began to decline rapidly, so much so that she needed hospice as well. She understood that she was now on her own journey and shared with me her desire for hospice care. But her family could not, and would not, let her go. They insisted that she seek aggressive treatment to cure what could not be cured. Hospitals and chemotherapy represented *their* only hope.

As I visited with her in the hospital one day, this wonderful woman confessed, "I just want to please them." We sat quietly for a while, and then she asked, "Ann, do you know the Twenty-third Psalm?"

"Yes, I do," I replied.

"Will you say it with me?"

"Of course, Lois."

The LORD is my shepherd, I shall not want;
    he makes me lie down in green pastures.
He leads me beside still waters;
    he restores my soul.
He leads me in paths of righteousness
    for his name's sake.
Even though I walk through the valley of the shadow
of death,
    I fear no evil;
for thou art with me;
    thy rod and thy staff,
    they comfort me.

Thou preparest a table before me
    in the presence of my enemies;
Thou anointest my head with oil,
    my cup overflows.
Surely goodness and mercy shall follow me
    all the days of my life;
And I shall dwell in the house of the LORD
    for ever. (RSV)

Lois, my unique and beautiful volunteer, died in a hospital, without the rewards of the hospice care she desired, the very hospice care she herself had given. And though, in the end, she set aside her wishes for those of her family, this was her choice. But she was not alone. Surrounding her bedside as she passed away was her immediate family and her hospice family.

Once, I worked with a volunteer whose son was dying of AIDS. She wanted to go through our training to decide if hospice care would be suitable for him. I made my assignments for her based on this motivation. Through the training and her hands-on experiences with patients, she learned of the hardships that lay ahead with her dying son.

What, then, are the benefits of having a volunteer on the hospice team? Though they are not professionals in the medical sense, volunteers are specialists in their desire to help. Unlike the nurse, the chaplain, or social worker, a volunteer arrives with no agenda. A volunteer rounds out this group by just *being there.*

As Cindy mentioned before, a caregiver can easily become overwhelmed with responsibilities. By being there, the volunteer is the ideal team member to respond to needs as simple, but as vital, as a trip to the grocery store. Being there, a caregiver is afforded an opportunity to leave troubles behind for a while and enjoy an uninterrupted lunch with a friend, a walk around the neighborhood, or the freedom to attend Sunday worship.

Sometimes a volunteer will be a better fit for the family if they are assigned to a family *member* instead of a patient. I recall another family whose son was dying of AIDS. Larry had not been home in a very long while; but now, he had come home to die. His mother, Sarah, and father, Jack, were in denial of his impending death, and the fact that *their* son had AIDS. No one else even knew he was dying.

The kitchen became Sarah's haven, while Jack lost himself in his woodshop. To further complicate matters, their long-awaited retirement plans would now have to be put on hold. The trailer in which they had expected to traverse the countryside now sat as a daily reminder of the disruption that their son represented.

Kay, a long-term volunteer, was assigned to the family. After assessing the situation, Kay determined that she could best serve Sarah. Once a week, Kay began to meet with her. They met for lunch, sometimes at a restaurant, sometimes in the local park. During the holidays, they met at the mall, talked, and watched the shoppers.

Kay could not change the fact that their son had AIDS. She could not, and would not, make Sarah or Jack face their feelings. But Kay became a touchstone for Sarah. Not only was Kay *there* for her, she *listened,* without judgment, as Sarah expressed her anger, frustration, resentment, and fear. It was all she could do. It was all she needed to do.

If you are ever to volunteer, remember the following:

When you make your first visit, you may feel anxious and fearful, honored and reverent, or a mixture of all these. You may feel a sense of immediacy. After all, someone is dying.

What can I do? you might ask yourself. It is important to understand that you do not necessarily need to *do* anything. From your training, you will be able to assess what a family or patient needs. Make no assumptions, and have no expectations before a visit.

As a volunteer, you are not expected to be an expert or a professional. Your role is to extend friendship and support. Do not be tempted to solve problems. Suggestions may be welcome, *but it is never appropriate to give advice.*

The idea is to relate to the *person,* not the illness. If a technical question is posed, it can always be deferred to another team member. Try to be aware of the family's ethics and values. If they differ from yours, it is not important that you agree with them. But it is important that you accept them. This is known as "unconditional positive regard." It conveys to the family that they are valued, no matter what.

Most of the time, just being there is enough. Often, it is your presence and not your words that mean the most. Perhaps the most important thing for you to do is to assess when a patient family wants to be left alone. Take your lead from them. And when you leave, set up your next visit, thereby reassuring the family of your availability.

Finally: You are walking into someone's life and death. You have come to offer what you can, and all that you can. You may never have met this family, and yet you are here. Be yourself. And God bless you. You are a volunteer.

CHAPTER TEN

In the End

John, Cindy, and Denise

A Prayer for Today

This is the beginning of a new day. God has given me this day to use as I will. I can waste it—or use it for good, but what I do today is important because I am exchanging a day of my life for it! When tomorrow comes, this day will be gone forever, leaving in its place something I have traded for it. I want it to be gain, and not loss; good, and not evil; success, and not failure, in order that I shall not regret the price that I have paid for it.

Author Unknown

For some time now, I have wondered which experience was more profound, the birth of my children or the death of my father. This seems like an odd comparison, I'm sure. One event is so happy and full of promise, and the other so painful and final. And if you believe the answer is obvious, then you have never lost someone you love. To me, this is worth thinking about.

But just as the daily growth of my children represents a part of my future, not a day goes by that I don't think of my dad and what was. He died two years ago, but only recently have I fully comprehended just how much his passing continues to impact my life, and that it always will. Ironically, this is the wondrous and beautiful thing about death. In this sense, it is not so final after all.

As physicians used all their medical science to prolong his life, I remember thinking that out of our technology has emerged the term *patient advocate.* In such a civilized country, why would any patient need an advocate?

The term would seem to imply that the tremendous advances of our society lack heart. What good does it serve us to have an open mind but a closed heart? In a time when we must ask permission to be allowed to die naturally, think of those who work in hospice as the ultimate patient advocates.

I think part of our problem today is that we have become too preoccupied with the world. And in this world, no one reaches the end of life unscathed. We all experience little deaths throughout our lives: thoughtless gestures or words, lost opportunities, failed relationships. Over time, it is easy to develop calluses on our hearts.

The pain we conceal is, nevertheless, pain we feel. To be a stranger to your emotions is to be a stranger to yourself. We need to look each other in the eyes more, touch each other more, and open our hearts to each other every day. Only then are we truly alive. It is our relationships with our fellow human beings, not our technology and entertainment, that make life worth living. This kind of intimacy is what gives our deaths meaning.

Denise, Cindy, Ann, Shelley, and Bobby, and all those working in hospice, face a daunting task. They seek nothing less than to change our culture. This is what must be done if we are to reclaim the true spirit of the death and dying experience.

Death is too intense an experience to be easy, or easily understood. I believe this is by design. But we make it harder than it should be.

John

———

It is often said to me, "It takes a unique person to do this kind of work. God has a special place in heaven for people like you." As much as I hate to admit it (*because it might tarnish my halo?*), I do, in fact, work in hospice for selfish reasons. Yes, I want to help my fellow human beings, but I derive a certain affirmation from the fact that someone needs me so much, that I can make such a tremendous difference in such a short time.

In what other job would someone—someone I may have known for only a few short hours—bother to call me on the anniversary of their loved one's death just to thank me once again?

I'm a nurse. It's easy for me to charge in on my white horse, bringing the great gifts of my leadership abilities, knowledge, and experience, and take control of a chaotic situation. Yes, this is easy for me and I am comfortable here, efficient and productive. But I have boundaries too. My problem is that, if I am not careful, this can become *my* situation. And it isn't.

My need for personal affirmation acknowledged, I must say that I receive even greater satisfaction from knowing I have helped my patients and their families most by empowering *them*. Imparting crucial knowledge and teaching specific skills needed to handle impending death empowers *them* to take control of their circumstances.

My challenge, then, has been to provide care based on *their* needs and not mine. A nurse's objectivity is valuable, but this is not *my* loved one who is dying. Deep, raw emotions must always be factored in, and we must never, ever, judge or second-guess one who is struggling with life and death, that time for which there are no clear-cut answers. My role is simply to extend an educated, supportive, calm, and compassionate helping hand.

"Cindy, why on earth would you want to care for a dying person?" This is a question I am frequently asked. At first, I had no answer other than that my heart, perhaps my very soul, was drawn to it. I could not imagine doing anything else. Later, I asked myself the same question. Why? Why did I feel so comfortable with this, when others naturally shied away? Why did I feel so rewarded, so fulfilled, so enriched and rejuvenated performing the mission of hospice?

The answer occurred to me one day as I was asked this question for what seemed the hundredth time.

"How can I not?" I replied. "I cannot imagine another field where I learn so much. These patients, whose lives I am *privileged* to enter, give me far more than I could ever hope to repay in kind. They teach me about myself, forcing me to look at life from perspectives I would probably never otherwise have considered."

I wish for you this difficult, joyous, painful, and unforgettable experience of helping another human being *live his or her life and death* in an atmosphere of unconditional love and acceptance. Even when, despite our best efforts, the experience is more painful than joyous, we have the comforting knowledge that we did our utmost to ensure a peaceful death.

As Elisabeth Kübler Ross once said, "And we learn, and we learn, and with each goodbye we learn."

Cindy

———

My experiences working in hospice are my stories. And my stories express as well as anything how and why I feel the way I do about my vocation. My intent is to show you that, no matter how grim it may seem, death should not to be feared. My last stories are of Ted and Lorraine.

Ted was a Vietnam veteran, a tough man who had seen death before. Here he was, at the young age of 42, unable to walk or sit up straight because his cancer was winning. A tumor the size of a football emerged from his neck, and the festering wound emitted a very foul smell. He did not want to die and leave his wife and children. But he had no choice in this matter.

On the last day of his life, I received a call from his family at 3:45 a.m. After I arrived, his parents, his wife, and I encircled his hospital bed, which was in the living room. I remember that it was dark, only one small lamp was turned on. They spoke of how much they loved him and how they would miss him. I spoke of God's love and mercy and told him that it was okay to let go.

His wife stroked his forehead and said, "I love you." Struggling for breath, he looked up at her. Then he said, "I love you too." Within moments, he died.

Death comes so quickly. We are seldom ready. Ted did want not die, but he was prepared, as was his family. This is where hospice is so valuable. For those who work in hospice, this is where we find our value, even fulfillment. We were able to be a part of that sacred time when a person passes from this life into the next. I was very honored that his family had asked me to share that moment.

Lorraine was dying of congestive heart failure. No longer able to live alone, she resided with her daughter, Patty. It was a cold autumn afternoon, and the wind was blowing as it does so often in Oklahoma. I remember so well sitting at the foot of her bed as Patty sat at her side and held her hand.

"You've been such a wonderful mother," she said softly, and began to stroke her mother's hair. "I love you so much. Don't worry about me. I'll be just fine. It's okay to die. Try to feel God's presence, God's love, and let go."

As she talked to her mother, I prayed silently for her journey from this life to the next. Patty continued to stroke her hair and tell her how much she loved her. When Lorraine drew her last breath, an immense feeling of love filled the room. It was a tangible thing; I could actually feel it.

Patty looked at me and said, "Thank you. I don't know what I would have done if it hadn't been for hospice."

I have tried to convey just how sacred these moments are, but words simply are not sufficient. I believe that at these moments, we stand on holy ground. Yes, death is hard. We do not want our loved ones to leave us. But hospice can provide a way for this journey to be one filled with love and dignity for all involved.

Elisabeth Kübler-Ross writes, "Those who have the strength and the love to sit with a dying patient *in the silence that goes beyond words* will know that this moment is neither frightening nor painful, but a peaceful cessation of the functioning of the body."[1]

We hope that this book will equip you with the tools and knowledge necessary to deal with death in a healthy way. We believe it is possible to make an unbearable situation bearable if we know what to do. This is why hospice is so important; it teaches us that death is a process and a journey, one that all will make.

I would like to leave with you this thought.

All we can really do is try to love each other and forgive each other. In doing so, maybe we can fulfill God's wish for us and *live* each moment.

And when life comes to an end, perhaps the kindest thing we can do is to be there, in whatever capacity we can, holding our loved one's hands as they walk this sacred journey.

Amen.

Denise

---

[1]Elisabeth Kübler-Ross, *On Death and Dying* (New York: Macmillan Publishing, 1969), p. 246.

Some There Are Who by Their Living

Some there are who by their living
    lift us to a higher plane,
finding joy disclosed in sorrow,
    healing hidden in their pain.
They are drawn by brighter visions,
    glad to give all they possess
for a greater good, discovering
    holier depths of happiness.

Some there are who by their dying
    lead us far beyond our fears,
showing us by their compassion
    hatred washed away by tears.
When contempts that we inherit
    fill us with hostility,
we have hope because of persons
    who have known love's liberty

Some there are who by their dying
    draw us closer to the Light,
finding death a blessed journey
    into that most gracious night.
When we feel the sting of knowing
    that our days are brief and swift,
we remember those whose living
    met each moment as a gift.

Thanks to God for those inviting
    us to live more faithfully!
Thanks to God for those who show us
    richer lives of charity!
Thanks for those we see no longer,
    but whose mem'ries in us lie!
Thanks to God for those who teach us
    how to live and how to die!

This hymn text was written by David L. Edwards, a Disciples of Christ minister, during the dying and deaths of his parents in 1993. It is lovingly dedicated to his parents, the Rev. B. P. and Ruby S. Edwards. The hymn in its original musical setting (Greencastle) may be found in *Chalice Hymnal* (St. Louis: Chalice Press, 1995), #648. Words © David L. Edwards, 1992. Reprinted by permission.

Appendix A

Values History Form

Name_____ Date_____

If someone assisted you in completing this form, please fill in his or her name, address, and relationship to you. Later on, it may be helpful to know more about your thought processes.

Name _____

Address _____

Relationship_____

The purpose of this form is to assist you in thinking about and writing down what is important to you about your health. If you should at some time become unable to make health care decisions for yourself, your thoughts as expressed on this form may help others make a decision for you in accordance with what you would have chosen.

The first section of this form asks whether you have already expressed your wishes concerning medical treatment through either written or oral communications and if not, whether you would like to do so now. The second section of this form provides an opportunity for you to discuss your values, wishes, and preferences in a number of different areas,

The Values History Form was developed by the Center for Health, Law, and Ethics in the Institue of Public Law, School of Law, University of New Mexico, Albuquerque, New Mexico (505/ 277–5006), and is reproduced by permission. Copies of this form may be made for personal use.

such as your personal relationships, your overall attitude toward life, and your thoughts about illness.

After you have completed this form, you may wish to provide copies to your doctors and other health caregivers, your family, your friends, and your attorney, If you have a Living Will, advance directive, or durable power of attorney for health care decisions, you may wish to attach a copy of this form to those documents.

SECTION ONE

A. WRITTEN LEGAL DOCUMENTS

Have you written any of the following legal documents?
❏ Yes   ❏ No
If so, please complete the requested information.

Living Will
Date written:_____
Document location: _____

Durable Power of Attorney
Date written: _____
Document location: _____
Comments: (e.g., whom have you named to be your decision maker?) _____
_____

Durable Power of Attorney for Health Care Decisions
Date written: _____
Document location: _____
Comments: (e.g., whom have you named to be your decision maker?) _____
_____

Organ Donations

Date written: _____

Document location: _____

Comments: (e.g., whom have you named to be your decision maker?) _____

B. Wishes Concerning Specific Medical Procedures

If you have ever expressed your wishes, either written or
orally, concerning any of the following medical procedures,
please complete the requested information. If you have not
previously indicated your wishes on these procedures and
would like to do so now, please complete this information.

Organ Donation

To whom expressed: _____

If oral, when?_____

If written, when? _____

Document location: _____

Comments: _____

Kidney Dialysis

To whom expressed: _____

If oral, when?_____

If written, when? _____

Document location: _____

Comments: _____

Cardiopulmonary Resuscitation (CPR)

To whom expressed: _____

If oral, when?_____

If written, when? _____

Document location: _____
Comments: _____
_____

Respirators

To whom expressed: _____
If oral, when? _____
If written, when? _____
Document location: _____
Comments: _____
_____

Artificial Nutrition

To whom expressed: _____
If oral, when? _____
If written, when? _____
Document location: _____
Comments: _____
_____

Artificial Hydration

To whom expressed: _____
If oral, when? _____
If written, when? _____
Document location: _____
Comments: _____
_____

C. GENERAL COMMENTS

Do you wish to make any general comments about the information you provided in this section?

SECTION TWO

A. YOUR OVERALL ATTITUDE TOWARD YOUR HEALTH

1. How would you describe your current health status?

   If you currently have any medical problems, how would you describe them?

2. If you have current medical problems, in what ways, if any, do they affect your ability to function?

3. How do you feel about your current health status?

4. How well are you able to meet the basic necessities of life: eating, food preparation, sleeping, personal hygiene, etc.?

5. Do you wish to make any general comments about your overall health?

B. YOUR PERCEPTION OF THE ROLE OF YOUR DOCTOR AND OTHER HEALTH CAREGIVERS

1. Do you like your doctors?

2. Do you trust your doctors?

3. Do you think your doctors should make the final decision concerning any treatment you might need?

4. How do you relate to your caregivers, including nurses, therapists, chaplains, social workers, etc.?

5. Do you wish to make any general comments about your doctor and other health caregivers?

C. YOUR THOUGHTS ABOUT INDEPENDENCE AND CONTROL

1. How important is independence and self-sufficiency in your life?

2. If you were to experience decreased physical and mental abilities, how would that affect your attitude toward independence and self-sufficiency?

3. Do you wish to make any general comments about the value of independence and control in your life?

D. Your Personal Relationships

1. Do you expect that your friends, family and/or others will support your decisions regarding medical treatments you may need now or in the future?

2. Have you made any arrangements for your family or friends to make medical treatment decisions on your behalf?

   If so, who has agreed to make decisions for you and in what circumstances?

3. What, if any, unfinished business from the past are you concerned about (e.g., personal and family relationships, business and legal matters)?

4. What role do your friends and family play in your life?

5. Do you wish to make any general comments about the personal relationships in your life?

E. Your Overall Attitude Toward Life

1. What activities do you enjoy (e.g., hobbies, watching TV, etc.)?

2. Are you happy to be alive?

3. Do you feel that life is worth living?

4. How satisfied are you with what you have achieved in the past?

5. What makes you laugh or cry?

6. What do you fear most?

   What frightens or upsets you?

7. What goals do you have for the future?

8. Do you wish to make any general comments about your attitude toward life?

F. YOUR RELIGIOUS BACKGROUND AND BELIEFS
   1. What is your religious background?

   2. How do your religious beliefs affect your attitude toward serious or terminal illness?

   3. Does your attitude toward death find support in your religion?

4. How does your faith community, church, or synagogue view the role of prayer or religious sacraments in an illness?

5. Do you wish to make any general comments about your religious background and beliefs?

G. YOUR LIVING ENVIRONMENT

1. What has been your living situation over the last ten years (e.g., lived alone, lived with others, etc.)?

2. How difficult is it for you to maintain the kind of environment for yourself that you find comfortable?

Does any illness or medical problem you now have mean that this will be harder in the future?

3. Do you wish to make any general comments about your living environment?

H. YOUR ATTITUDE CONCERNING FINANCES

    1. How much do you worry about having enough money to provide for your care?

    2. Would you prefer to spend less money on your care so that more money can be saved for the benefit of your relatives and/or friends?

    3. Do you wish to make any general comments concerning your finances and the cost of health care?

I. YOUR WISHES CONCERNING YOUR FUNERAL

    1. What are your wishes concerning your funeral and burial or cremation?

    2. Have you made your funeral arrangements?

    If so, with whom?

3. Do you wish to make any general comments about how you would like your funeral and burial or cremation to be arranged and conducted?

J. OTHER QUESTIONS TO CONSIDER

1. How would you like your obituary (announcement of your death) to read?

2. Write yourself a brief eulogy (a statement about yourself to be read at your funeral).

Appendix B

Universal Precautions

Universal precautions are used to prevent the transmission of disease from one person to another. They are based on the idea of preventing any comingling of body fluids (in other words, keeping each person's body fluids from touching the other person's body fluids). This listing is not intended to be all-inclusive, but rather to highlight fundamental concepts of practicing universal precautions.

1. *Always assume everyone has a potentially dangerous infection, such as HIV or hepatitis, that can be passed on to you.* This is what is meant by *Universal* Precautions—we universally assume *everyone* has an infection and act accordingly.

2. *Always wear the appropriate personal protective equipment (PPE) needed to prevent exposure to body fluids.* What is appropriate will depend upon the situation. Sometimes just latex gloves are enough, such as when emptying a urinal. If the person has lost control of bladder or bowels and clean-up is likely to be extensive, a gown *and* gloves may be required.

3. *Practice good hand-washing.* Wash before *and* after touching the person, and before applying make-up; after sneezing, coughing, and using the bathroom; and before handling contact lenses. Scrub your hands for at least twenty seconds, using an antimicrobial (germkilling) soap. Wearing gloves does *not* mean you don't have to wash your hands—wash every time you remove gloves. If it feels as if you are washing your

hands a hundred times a day—you're probably washing enough.

4. Follow these steps to clean up any spills of blood or body fluids:

- Clean up body substances right away.
- Get a plastic bag for disposal of paper towels.
- Wipe up the spill with paper towels.
- Use more towels to clean the surface with hot water and soap or detergent.
- Rinse all soap or detergent from the surface.
- Apply a bleach and water solution of 10% bleach to 90% water.
- Leave it on the surface for 10 minutes, then wipe dry.
- Put latex gloves in the bag.
- Seal the bag, and place it in a second plastic bag for disposal.
- Disinfect utility gloves in bleach and water.

5. *Clothing and linens soiled with body fluids should be laundered in detergent and the hottest water safe for the fabric.* Bleach added to the load will also help with controlling the spread of infection.

Appendix C

Relieving the Dis-Ease of Stress

Bobbie Crabb Jennings

Exercises

These exercises can be used by almost anyone, any place, and in most any position: sitting, lying down, or standing. They are designed to assist with relaxation and pain management. They will also help maintain the "range of motion" of the joints, slow down the wasting of muscle, and improve blood flow. Most importantly, they provide active participation and empowerment, even if all an individual can do is to take in a deep, cleansing breath while the caretaker gently moves an arm or leg.

Never force movement into a painful range. Remember, a person in pain will tense up, and this may trigger the pain cycle. Any of these exercises that cannot be performed independently because of pain, mental status, or weakness can be done with assistance. But keep in mind, always *exercise* caution, never force a movement.

Exercises that involve any type of rotary action (movement caused by force) of the bones might cause stress fractures. Avoid these types of exercises because loss of bone mass accompanies prolonged illnesses.

For those patients who cannot perform exercises on their own, it is absolutely necessary that you discuss any exercise with a healthcare professional beforehand.

1. Shoulder rolls: Slowly lift shoulders toward ears, then slowly roll shoulders back as you gently pinch shoulder blades together. BREATHE! Repeat 2 times.
2. Shoulder shrugs: Again, slowly lift shoulders toward ears. Hold to a count of 5 while taking a deep breath. Bring them back to normal position. Repeat 2 times.
3. Neck rotations: Slowly rotate chin to left shoulder—hold to a count of 3 while taking a deep breath. Rotate to the right, as you did to the left. Repeat 2 times.
4. Chin tucks: Slowly bring chin toward chest. Hold to a count of 5 while taking a deep breath. Return to neutral. Repeat 2 times.
5. Side bends: Attempt to place left ear on left shoulder, slowly. Hold to a count of 3. Repeat on right side. Return to neutral. Repeat 2 times.
6. Buttocks pinches: Breathing slowly and deeply, pull in your stomach muscles while pinching your buttocks together. Hold to the count of 4. Repeat 2 times.
7. Quad sets: Breathing slowly and deeply, with legs straight, gently lock both knees and hold to the count of 3. Repeat 5 times.
8. Ankle pumps/circles: As you take in a deep breath, slowly pull your toes toward your knees. Exhale slowly and push toes toward the ground. Make a circle with your big toes. Repeat 5 times with each ankle.
9. Arm lifts: As you take in a deep breath, bend one knee and bring toward chin. Exhale slowly and return leg to straightened position. Repeat 2 times with each leg.
10. Leg bends: As you take in a deep breath, bend one knee and bring toward your chin. Exhale slowly and return the leg to a straightened position. Repeat 2 times with each leg.
11. Windshield wipers: With legs straight and apart, slowly roll knees and hips in, then out. Your feet become windshield wipers! Repeat 2 times on each leg.

Remember: Deep breathing is used to ease pain. Slowly breathe in through your nose and out through your mouth as you perform each exercise.

Massage

Stress and pain cause muscle tension. This, in turn, leads to spasms and knots commonly found in the neck and back. Muscle tension is a major factor in the pain cycle, so relieving tension often relieves pain. There are several types of massage, from light stroking to deep kneading. If not performed correctly, this could be harmful to those with conditions such as blood clots, cancer, and osteoporosis.

It is wise to consult a medical professional before performing anything beyond a light touch or gentle stroking massage. Following a bath, a gentle massage can be given as body lotions and powders are applied. Lotion or powder allows the hands to flow across the skin with less friction and can make the massage much more pleasant.

It is absolutely necessary that the massage *does not* create pain or discomfort. Some individuals do not want to be touched. *Undesired touching can cause increased tension and stress.* Always ask permission before you touch anyone.

Appendix D

Positioning

There comes a time when exercise is not possible. Therefore, you should be aware of *positioning*. When positioning a patient in bed for any length of time, special care must be taken to avoid bedsores. A person who is incapable of moving independently in bed should *never* be left for more than two hours in any one position. If the person is fragile and thin, one hour should be the limit. Comfort is the main goal, but postural alignment, function, and safety must also be considered. Many pillows are required!

Every time the patient is repositioned, the skin must be inspected for redness–most especially those sections that are in contact with *bony* areas. If the redness does not go away within thirty minutes, do not return the patient to that position for 24 hours. Be sure other caregivers are aware of this. Bedsores are caused from pressure and can be prevented with careful, consistent inspection by all caregivers.

If a person is in severe pain, frequent position changes often help. When repositioning, avoid *grabbing* the muscles. Rather, lift arms and legs under the joints, or support a body part with your forearms as you move it. Always roll patients toward you, pulling from the back of their shoulder and hip. Ask the person to help as much as possible, because this will help keep muscle toned.